BUILDING SPELLING SKILLS
in dyslexic children

Edited by John I. Arena

Assisted by Bonnie Harrington

ACADEMIC THERAPY PUBLICATIONS
San Rafael, California 94901

©

About the Authors . . .

MARTHA S. AHO

Mrs. Aho is a fourth-grade teacher in the Highlands School, Renton, Washington. She has worked closely with Mrs. Beth Slingerland in conducting programs employing the Slingerland adaptation of the Orton-Gillingham multisensory approach for teaching children who have specific language disability.

BERNARD BAILEY

Mr. Bailey has taught at the elementary-school level in the Minnesota public schools. He is at present doing graduate work at the University of Wisconsin, Madison.

HELEN S. BARNETTE

Mrs. Barnette is director of reading for the Oil City, Pennsylvania, Area Schools. She has a background in classroom teaching, kindergarten through college levels, as well as in remedial teaching. She has also served as a reading consultant.

HAROLD BLAU

Mr. Blau is director of the (L.I.) Reading and Tutoring Insitute, Inc., a learning center and school in Jamaica, New York. He is the author of *How to Write the College Entrance Exam "Writing Sample"* (Philadelphia, Penn.: Chilton, n.d.). He is preparing for his doctorate at the New York University School of Education.

BLAKE K. BROWNE

Mr. Browne has taught at the elementary-school level in the Wisconsin public schools. He is now a tutor of learning-disabled children in the Chicago, Illinois, area.

ROBERT K. BRUCE

Mr. Bruce was a private remedial consultant in Boston, Massachusetts. He has also taught at the elementary-school level in the New England area. He is now doing private remedial work on the Pacific Coast.

LEE CRAWFORD

Mrs. Crawford is executive director of the Edgemoor School, Houston, Texas. She has served as legislative chairman of the Council for Exceptional Children, as chairman for the Professional Directory of the Texas Association for Children with Learning Disabilities, as corresponding secretary of Houston A.C.L.D., convention chairman for T.A.C.L.D., and as a member of the A.C.L.D. nominating committee. She is the author of a series of seven booklets on learning disabilities, including *Perceptual Motor and Learning* and *The Importance of Discipline* (Houston, Tex.: Edgemoor Publications). These booklets are available through A.C.L.D. chapters in the United States and Canada, as well as in some European countries.

PHYLLIS W. DOLE

Mrs. Dole is director of educational planning for Hoffman Information Systems, a division of Hoffman Electronics, Riverside, California. She has a background as a classroom teacher in elementary school and as a remedial-reading teacher. She established the first Instructional Materials Center for the Riverside Unified Schools and was director of the program for two years. She has served in the administrative capacity of vice-principal and principal of several schools and was director of the Learning Center, Riverside, California, a learning disabilities clinic established under Title III funding.

RUTH EDGINGTON

Mrs. Edgington is an education specialist at the Child Study Center, University of Arkansas Medical Center, Little Rock. She has twenty-one years experience as a teacher of special education, has instructed in summer teachers' courses, has served as an educational consultant, and has been active in many parent and professional organizations concerned with learning disabilities. She is a contributing

i

editor to *Academic Therapy* and has made a number of significant contributions to the literature of learning disabilities, including, with Sam D. Clements, an *Indexed Bibliography on the Educational Management of Children with Learning Disabilities* (Chicago, Ill.: Argus Communications, 1967).

EULA FARNHAM
Mrs. Farnham is a private tutor and reading and learning therapist in Santa Fe, New Mexico. She has a background of classroom teaching, kindergarten through college levels, as well as in remedial work.

PETER GLUSKER
Mr. Glusker is a research assistant in the Program in Biological Psychology, University of Oklahoma Medical Center, Oklahoma City. He was formerly an academic therapist with the DeWitt Reading Clinic, San Rafael, California, and served as a visiting research worker at the Oxford Institute of Experimental Psychology.

HAROLD B. HELMS
Mr. Helms has taught at the elementary and junior-high-school levels and is now an academic therapist with the DeWitt Reading Clinic, San Rafael, California. He received his M.A. from the University of California, Berkeley, and is doing graduate work at that institution.

HOMER HENDRICKSON
Dr. Hendrickson, an optometrist in Temple City, California, is associate director and Western Zone chairman of the Section on Children's Vision Care and Guidance of the Optometric Extension Program. He has served as secretary of the California Optometric Association, chairman of the board of trustees of the Los Angeles College of Optometrists (1959-65), and was named Optometrist of the Year in 1960 by the California Optometric Association. He has written extensively on visual development and skill in relation to learning, including a chapter, with G. N. Getman, on "The Needs of Teachers for Specialized Information on the Development of Visuo-Motor Skills in Relation to Academic Performance," which appeared in *The Teacher of Brain-Injured Children*, ed. William M. Cruickshank (Syracuse, N.Y.: Syracuse University Press, 1966).

JEFFREY L. HICKS
Mr. Hicks is a doctoral candidate in school psychology at the University of Oregon in Eugene. During 1967-68 he held a fellowship in the Education of Exceptional Children at the University of Oregon, and he is a member of Psi Chi, a national academic honorary society in psychology.

KATIE G. HIGGINS
Miss Higgins is a remedial consultant and private tutor in Los Angeles, California. Her background includes teaching regular as well as special classes in California and Oregon schools. She received her M.A. from the University of Hawaii.

GERALDINE M. KIMMELL
Mrs. Kimmell is director of the Reading Laboratories at Marin Country Day School for the DeWitt Reading Clinic, San Rafael, California.

BRIAN LATTIMORE
Mr. Lattimore has taught at the elementary, junior-high, and senior-high-school levels in Upper New York State. He received his M.A. from the University of Oregon, Eugene.

RAYMOND E. LAURITA
Mr. Laurita recently received an N.D.E.A. College Teaching Fellowship for doctoral study at State University of New York, Albany. He was formerly a reading specialist with the Schroon Lake Central and Moriah Central Schools and has an extensive background of classroom and remedial teaching. He is a member of the National Advisory Council of the Reading Reform Foundation, and he recently presented a workshop on reading at the Lake George Conference on Learning Disabilities presented by the School Psychologists of New York State. His contributions to the literature of learning and teaching have appeared in many popular and professional journals and include: "Phonics vs. Look-Say: Is the End in Sight?" *N.Y.S. Education* (March 1967); "Does Keeping a Child Back Help or Hinder?" *Crisis* (September 1967); and "Errors Children Make in Reading," *Spelling Progress Bulletin* (Fall 1967).

ELLWOOD C. LILLY
Mr. Lilly is a teacher in the Los Angeles City Schools and president of the Foundation for Developmental Teaching, Inc., Van Nuys, California. He is also doing graduate work at the University of Southern California.

SHIRLEY H. LINN
Mrs. Linn is a teacher for the Perceptual Training Program in Kindergarten with the Topeka, Kansas, Unified School District. In addition to having experience as a regular classroom teacher, she has been a teacher of the homebound, and taught the first class for neurologically impaired children in the state

of Kansas. She has also been a visiting lecturer at Texas Woman's University. She is particularly interested in the identification and remediation of the early symptoms of learning disorders.

BETTY D. MADISON

Mrs. Madison, in addition to teaching educationally handicapped children at the Springhill School, Lafayette, California, acts as a consultant and workshop leader for various school districts and as a guest lecturer for organizations. Her background includes duties as director of a nursery school and as an elementary-school teacher. Among her published works is "A Framework for Reading," which appeared in *Teaching Educationally Handicapped Children* (San Rafael, Calif.: Academic Therapy Publications, 1967). She received her A.B. from the University of California, Berkeley, and has continued her studies at that institution and at San Francisco State College.

RONALD J. McEWAN

Mr. McEwan, former director of the Napa, California, branch of the DeWitt Reading Clinic, is now a teacher of the educationally handicapped in the Healdsburg, California, Junior High School. He received his B.A. from San Francisco State College.

MICHAEL G. POWERS

Mr. Powers is a private tutor and remedial therapist in the San Francisco Bay Area. He received his M.A. from the University of Utah.

LYLE PUTNAM

Mr. Putnam has taught classes of educationally handicapped children in Northern California and is now a private remedial tutor in the Sacramento, California, area. He received his B.A. from Denver (Colorado) University.

SARAH A. SHAFER

Mrs. Shafer is a teacher in the Los Angeles City Schools and executive vice-president of the Foundation for Developmental Teaching, Inc., Van Nuys, California. She is doing graduate work at the University of California, Los Angeles.

BICKLEY F. SIMPSON

Mrs. Simpson is at present the associate research director of Laboratory Schools for Children, Lesley College, Cambridge, Massachu-

setts. In 1969, she will assume the duties of project director under a Learning Disabilities Grant at Lesley College. She was formerly an associate at Perceptual Education and Research Center, Lesley College, and a member of the graduate faculty at that institution. She is the author of *Project Lighthouse Training Kit* (in press) and a candidate for the Ed. D. in communications disorders at Boston University.

ROSALYN TAUBER

Miss Tauber is a learning-disabilities specialist with the Summit, New Jersey, Public Schools and a speech and reading clinician with the New York Infirmary, Child Guidance Clinic, New York City. She was formerly a tester in a research project, evaluating speech, hearing, and language development, at Columbia Presbyterian Medical Center, and a coordinator and teacher in speech and hearing services, Livingston, New Jersey, Public Schools. Among her published works in the field of learning disabilities are, "Identification of Potential Learning Disabilities," *Academic Therapy Quarterly,* II (Winter 1967); and "The Child Study Team," *N.J.E.A. Review,* XXXVIII (May 1965). She received her M.A. from Columbia University and has taken postgraduate training at that institution and at the College of the City of New York.

JACK WAHL

Mr. Wahl, an academic therapist at the DeWitt Reading Clinic, San Rafael, California, directs projects for the DeWitt Research Center for Academic Development. He received his M.A. from San Francisco State College.

NELDA WARWICK

Mrs. Warwick is an independent consultant to school districts in the Southern California area. She received her M.A. from the University of California at Goleta.

SANDRA WINKLER

Miss Winkler was formerly an elementary-school teacher in the San Francisco Public Schools. She has a background in private tutorial and remedial work. She received her B.A. from the University of Washington.

WILLIAM W. WULPE

Mr. Wulpe has taught learning-disabled children in various private schools and clinics in the New York City area. He is at present doing private remedial work. He received his M.A. from New York University.

INTRODUCTION

THE EXPERIENCE of many teachers and parents suggests that some children are natural spellers. They usually spell words correctly once they are learned and, when they do make a mistake, one correction is generally sufficient. They have developmentally acquired the organizational skills of integration necessary to learn to spell efficiently.

The fact that there are youngsters who are spelling-competent makes it difficult to understand the failure of others, many of whom seem to be as alert, intelligent, and capable as those who are succeeding. Many parents, teachers, and remedial specialists recognize that the underachieving child is not necessarily dull, lazy, spoiled, resistive, or indifferent. Frequently the youngster is just as frustrated as is the person trying to help him. He desperately wants to be able to spell, but simply cannot seem to get the letters onto the paper in the correct order or without substituting, adding, or omitting letters.

Out of this recognition has grown the awareness that there are potentially capable children who are not able (or ready) to learn to spell by traditional educational methods. It is fairly obvious that the old method of "write it ten times" is not an outstanding success, as witnessed by the many young people who reach college age and adulthood while still plagued with serious spelling deficiencies.

Out of need grows innovation – and many individuals and organizations working with underachieving children have, through innovation, found ways of helping the child to learn in his own unique way, utilizing the sensory modalities through which that child learns most effectively.

In response to many requests received over a two-year period for remedial approaches specifically geared to helping children overcome spelling deficiencies, the Fall 1967 issue of *Academic Therapy* was devoted entirely to this subject. Following publication, the demand for additional copies of the special issue by parents, organizations, and remedial specialists from many fields emphasized the need for a still more comprehensive compilation and one that would be available on a continuing basis.

Building Spelling Skills in Dyslexic Children is such a compilation. The children needing help and the reasons for their failure to learn are unique and varied – as are the physical conditions in which they are to be taught. With this in mind, new articles were added to those that appeared in the special issue of *Academic Therapy* with the aim of presenting a wide variety of adaptable and versatile approaches. The articles suggest means of developing and reinforcing the under-lying perceptual and academic skills necessary for competent spelling. They are directed to those remedial workers who are searching for creative approaches beyond the usual routine assignments and weekly spelling tests, in order to meet the challenge of teaching children to spell – children who, although intellectually capable, are unable to learn by conventional methods.

Those who have so generously participated in this compilation offer what they have found to be of help, in both public and private academic settings, in leading their students to greater achievement. Their diversified viewpoints are presented so that the reader may evaluate, select, and adapt in a way creatively suited to the needs of his own situation.

It is hoped that the ideas presented in *Building Spelling Skills* will be tried and expanded, perhaps leading to further innovation, to be shared, in turn, with others seeking ways of helping children to achieve up to their own fullest potential. It is our belief that this sharing is the strength of our educational system.

J. I. A.

CONTENTS

Unusual Measures for the Spelling Invalid

Harold Blau

FOR THE AFFLICTION known as extremely poor spelling, two new procedures may provide visible improvement in a reasonable period of time and, in some cases, almost complete relief. Generally found associated with serious reading deficiencies, poor spelling is, of course, not infrequently found among good readers also. In either case, treatment tends to take two forms:

- He needs basic drill; make him work.
- Penalize him and hope he gets over it.

Neither approach is distinguished for its profundity nor for more than occasional success.

The new procedures suggested here are: (1) A recording, writing, self-dictating method centered around a tape recorder, the object of which is to make the student himself into a kind of self-teaching device and part of a "responsive environment." (2) A nonvisual technique whereby the student, with eyes closed or blindfolded, "constructs" the troublesome words with three-dimensional letters and traces them with his finger while an aide prints the same letters in block form on his back. (The student is nearly always a "he," of course.)

THE TAPE RECORDER method is basically quite simple. The student gets ready to record his voice. He pronounces his first word into the microphone. With the tape recorder still running, he writes or copies the word twice, marks off the syllables, if any, says the word again, and spells it aloud. He does the same with the next word and the next for a total of five or ten words. Only at the very end does he shut off the tape recorder.

He now studies the words — hard parts, syllable parts, word-within-a-word parts, and so forth. Having done this, he dons his earphone and plays the whole thing back.

The earphone is extremely important. Not only does it prevent intruding on others with amplified sound, it also insures privacy. There is no embarrassment, therefore, for the student, and so no temptation to clown or otherwise to subvert the learning situation.

The student is his own teacher. His voice is the dominant one, rather than that of some teacher-authority associated only with failure. Copying the word twice gives him ample time to think when it comes to taking it by dictation, and the correct spelling coming at the end corrects mistakes — again, in complete privacy.

1

The student goes over the tape at least once in full, and then as often as may be deemed necessary to correct stubborn errors. The tape may be retained and, as material is added, a kind of spiral review process is also begun to insure mastery.

Of course, an aide is needed to help with the pronunciation of words and with the identification of syllable parts since the student usually cannot do this by himself.

IN THE METHOD where the eyes are closed or blindfolded, as indicated previously, the student says the word and calls off the letters as they are printed on his back by an aide. He has put the words together with three-dimensional letters and may touch or trace the letters if he is uncertain. After two (or more) practice runs, he must be able to say the letters only as he feels them. The three-dimensional letters are then scrambled and the student puts them together in proper sequence. If successful, he is permitted to take off the blindfold and to write the word two or three times on his paper or on the blackboard.

All in all, this is a slower method and it may have to be used on the same word more than once, but there seems to be no transition problem. Once the student masters a word with his eyes closed, he recognizes it in a normal manner when he meets it again.

NOW, why blindfolding? Why tracing? Why printing on the back? The answers are somewhat indirect. Everyone has read about, and some have practiced, closing the eyes to learn to spell. Everyone has heard of, and some have practiced, tracing letters to learn to read (the Fernald method).[1] In the method under discussion, the blindfolding is to make sure the eyes remain closed and the tracing is to provide letter and syllable recognition. The printing on the back has a number of purposes. It fills in the gap caused by the missing visual input (the teacher of the visually handicapped should be particularly alert to this), and it insures realization of letter sequence and directionality.

Interestingly, there seems to be a kind of folklore or subculture involving writing on the back that has not been noted heretofore but which will emerge wherever this technique is used. Parents will remember that they used it in games or that their mothers used it for "hard" spelling words.

Both techniques are completely individual and as such are not compatible with typical class routines. Individual tutors are needed, but these need not be more exalted than teacher internes, student aides, or, occasionally, the spelling invalids themselves working with each other.

For the student with whom "nothing has ever worked," these methods can evoke so much hope that caution and restraint must be the watchwords and moderation counseled until the actual rate of progress has been demonstrated.

In hard-core learning cases, with the blindfolding method, word recognition and reading also seem to benefit as modality conflict is eased.[2]

THREE QUESTIONS may require consideration. One is whether

[1] Harriet Blau and Harold Blau, "Some Multisensory Approaches for the Severely Disabled Reader," *Reading* (March 2, 1968), pp. 5-10.

[2] Harriet Blau, "Modality Blocking Technique." Paper delivered at the Fifth International Convention, Association for Children with Learning Disabilities, Boston, Massachusetts. February 3, 1968.

either method ever gets boring. The answer is, of course, just as anything else does if pursued without relief or variation. Retesting, charts of progress, checking on progress in the regular classroom, word games, material on word origins, crossword puzzles, and so forth, are as necessary for these students as they are for more normal situations. However, students seem to be able to work for longer periods of time before becoming bored, especially when using the tape recording method. There is the fascination of the toy for the child, the interest in the sound of one's own voice, and the sense of independent control — all of which serve to emancipate the student from the usual sense of the slow passage of time.

The second question is where to find the words that must be learned. So far as the writer is concerned this is not extremely important. One school of thought stresses the words the student himself wants to learn and this is probably reasonable. From the author's own experience, the most important consideration is that the words come from some organized material — a story, a composition, a television commercial, any paragraph of text — so that spelling is properly and unobtrusively reinforced by contextual use and meaning.

The third question is whether both methods may be used with the same student. The answer is, "Certainly."

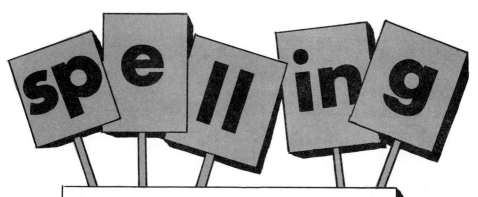

SIGN SPELLING is an excellent spelling game for rainy days when a class activity is needed. Letters are printed on pieces of six-by-ten-inch tagboard, one card for each child. The letters might be single consonants and vowels, a blend (*gr, bl, sl*), or syllables (*ack, ust, ame*). The children then take turns in selecting two or three other youngsters to come to the front of the room and placing them in the proper order to spell a word. The word is then written as a total unit on the chalkboard and one youngster is chosen to pronounce it.

Notes on Spelling Tests

Nelda Warwick

———————◆———————

FOR the classroom teacher, spelling tests basically have one major function: to test the achievement of the child. That is, how many words can the child spell when compared to other children in the same grade-age category? Unfortunately, an overlooked aspect of such spelling tests is their diagnostic value to the teacher or clinician.

By careful use of standardized achievement tests, teachers can learn a great deal about the spelling difficulties of the child, over and above the determination of a grade-equivalency score.

What we really want to learn from a spelling test is how well the child can translate into writing the words he uses in his reading and speaking vocabularies. Nonstandardized instruments, such as the weekly spelling tests, can also yield a wealth of information which can be used by the teacher to help the child. Following are some suggestions.

• How does the child compare with his classmates in the total number of words spelled correctly? This can be computed on a number-right–number-wrong basis or on a percentage basis, and a graph can be maintained, from week to week, by the child.

• What is the status of other written work prepared by the child? Are there continual errors in his written homework and written classroom assignments?

• When spelling tests over a period of time are evaluated, are there consistent kinds of errors? For example:

(a) Does the error usually involve the terminal sound; i.e., *had* for *hat*?

(b) Are syllables usually missing; i.e., *evning* for *evening* ?

(c) Are there inversions or misplacements of letters; i.e., *left* for *felt*?

(d) Are letters added; i.e., *lounch* for *lunch*?

• Are weekly tests generally good (eighty percent or better) and review tests poor (fifty percent or below)?

WHEN TESTS are carefully evaluated, the teacher may be able to arrive at some preliminary generalizations about the basic problems of the child and his needs for spelling improvement.

I remember two incidents which illustrate some pertinent points. One little girl, when she meant to spell *right*, spelled *rat* – however, this was the way she pronounced it. Another youngster spelled *that* as *dat* – again because this is the way he was able to say it.

While the evidence in both cases superficially suggests reinforcement in phonics, both illustrate different problems. The little girl was spelling the words correctly as she pronounced them. The boy had a subtle auditory discrimination problem and perceived the *th* sound as a *d*. Observing the language patterns of children is, therefore, a necessary ingredient in the total act of evaluating a spelling problem.

When a teacher wishes to obtain more formal information about the spelling ability of the students, either individually or in a group, specific tests are available. Following are some of them.

• There are spelling tests which are a part of a reading test. For example, the Durrell-Sullivan Achievement Test contains a spelling test of twenty words. In such a case, the teacher can obtain a spelling score and compare it to the reading score. (This test is for children in grades three through six and there are two forms, A and B.)

• The Wide Range Achievement Test has three parts; reading, arithmetic, and spelling. The spelling test may be given separately or as part of the total test and may be used with one child or a group of children. There are two levels, I and II, which are for those aged 11.11 and under and those above age 12.0. There are forty-six words in each level, but testing is discontinued when the child has missed ten words. There is only one form of the test. It yields a grade equivalent, a standard score, and a percentile.

• The Lincoln Diagnostic Spelling Test includes spelling only. It offers an intermediate form (grades five through eight) and an advanced form (grades nine through twelve), with A and B forms for both (which allows for retesting with different words). The test allows the teacher to break down errors into ten error categories, an aid for remedial programming. The sentences which are dictated by the examiner are printed on the answer sheet, and space is allowed in which the word is to be written. There are one hundred words in each form. Final scores are given in percentiles.

• The Phonovisual Diagnostic Spelling Test is designed for children in grades three and up. It is a "test for all consonant sounds and the seventeen fundamental vowel sounds," and is structured to discover phonetic weaknesses. There are twenty words in all and they are all one-syllable words. There is one form only of the test.

• The National Achievement Spelling Test contains four separate levels: grades three through four, grades five through eight, grades seven through nine, and grades ten through twelve. The child's test form contains the sentence to be dictated by the examiner but without the dictated word which is to be spelled by the child. A median grade-level score is yielded. The number of words varies from fifty on the lower forms to sixty on the higher forms.

• Often there is a need for a teacher to administer tests more frequently than once or twice a year. For this purpose the Buckingham Extension of the Ayres Spelling Scale is extremely useful. This scale is based on both the most commonly used words in written communication and words most commonly found in spellers. Teachers can create their own tests and obtain grade-equivalent scores by using the word lists given in the manual.

• For students in grades nine through twelve, the Traxler High School Spelling Test is a useful instrument, since three equivalent forms (1, 2, and 3) are available. Each of fifty

5

words (in each form) is dictated. The student's sheet contains a sentence for each word with a space in which the word is to be written. The examiner does not read the sentence; only the word is given. A value of the test is that it gives percentile ratings corresponding to scores of independent school pupils for each of the three forms.

OTHER TESTS are available and catalogues should be consulted. Most schools maintain an up-to-date file on published tests and, in many cases, the publishers will send, for a small fee, a specimen kit for examination.

Whether the teacher uses the "informal" or the "formal" test, she should always keep in mind the question: "How will this test help me to help the child?"

REFERENCES

Buckingham, B. R. *Buckingham Extension of the Ayres Spelling Scale* (Indianapolis, Ind.: Bobbs-Merrill, n.d.).

Durrell, Donald D., and Helen Sullivan. *Durrell-Sullivan Achievement Test* (New York: Harcourt, Brace and World, 1965).

Jastak, J. F., S. W. Bijou, and S. R. Jastak. *Wide Range Achievement Test* (Wilmington, Del.: Guidance Associates, 1965).

Lincoln, A. L. *Lincoln Diagnostic Spelling Test* (Indianapolis, Ind.: Bobbs-Merrill, 1956).

Schoolfield, Lucille D., and Josephine B. Timberlake. *Phonovisual Diagnostic Spelling Test* (Washington, D.C.: Phonovisual Products, 1949).

Speer, Robert K., and Samuel Smith. *National Achievement Spelling Test* (Rockville Centre, New York: Acorn Publishing Co., 1960; Chicago, Ill.: Psychometric Affiliates).

Traxler, Arthur E., *Traxler High School Spelling Test* (Indianapolis, Ind.: Bobbs-Merrill, 1955).

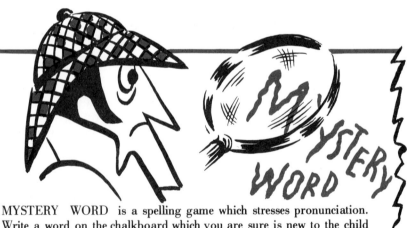

MYSTERY WORD is a spelling game which stresses pronunciation. Write a word on the chalkboard which you are sure is new to the child or the class. Have each child in turn try to pronounce the word. Write each child's interpretation of the word on the chalkboard as he gives it. When each child has had a chance to pronounce the word, tell the class what the correct pronunciation of the word is.

The next day, pass out a list of all the words that were presented and see how many of the children can correctly pronounce the words given on the previous day.

Teaching Spelling to Children with Specific Language Disability

Martha S. Aho

———————◆———————

A SEEMINGLY bright boy in my class, whose writing and spelling simply was not commensurate with his ability, complained, "I know how to spell that word but my hand just won't write it the way I want it to." Before I learned to understand his difficulty, I would have thought to myself: "Well, at least that excuse is different—but where am I falling short in meeting his needs? Others with much less ability seem to be making much more progress." Now I realize how much he was really telling me, because he was one of the ten to twenty per cent of the children found in our classrooms today who has a specific language disability.

Renton, Washington, was indeed fortunate the day that Mrs. Beth Slingerland joined the teaching staff of the public schools. Not only did she bring to us the knowledge of specific language disability and an understanding of this particular kind of failure (so we could stop blaming ourselves), but of even greater importance, she told us *how* these children could be taught—something for which many teachers had been groping for a long time.[1]

In gratitude for the opportunity I had to learn about S.L.D., which gave us a new approach to teaching, I would like to share with others the help I received from Mrs. Slingerland who has taught and patiently helped and guided so many for the past six years. I shall try to tell (1) how these children are identified, (2) how early identification and preventive training lessens the remediation necessary, and (3) how spelling may be taught to children with specific language disability.

Emphasis is first placed on early identification and placement in the proper program before an individual's problems become too complex. Screening tests, now published, are given to all children entering the first grade, new entrants, children in question, or when new groups are to be formed in schools for the first time.[2] Factors such as intelligence, family pattern of handedness, language difficulties in relatives, early speech delays, and teacher observations are closely related to the screening tests as evaluations are made.

The children who are identified as potential, borderline, to severe disability cases are placed in classroom groups, with trained teachers following a

---

[1] Teachers, seeking answers, prevailed upon Mrs. Slingerland for help. This led to summer-school sessions with college credit granted from Seattle Pacific College. Today Renton has many trained teachers working with hundreds of children in numerous elementary schools, some with classes from the first through the sixth grades. Besides local teachers, others have come for training from as far away as Alaska, Canada, California, Florida, New Jersey, and Texas.

[2] Beth Slingerland, *Screening Tests for Identifying Children with Specific Language Disability* (Cambridge, Mass.: Educators Publishing Service, 1964).

continuous pattern in technique through each level. The potential or borderline cases rarely show any signs of difficulty after two or three years of training and they move ahead with a feeling of success. They could go into regular classrooms as indicated by performance and achievement tests, but they, and their parents, usually prefer that they stay for further help as long as it can be given. The severe disability cases learn to cope with their difficulties, have good attitudes, and are most tolerant and understanding of others with the same weaknesses.

In contrast are the transfers who enter the program after failure has magnified negative attitudes and loss of self-confidence. They react in many ways— apathetic, anxious, depressed, and sometimes even hostile or rebellious. When encouragement is offered by others about them with the same difficulties, a surprising improvement in effort, attitude, and self-enhancement is noticed. Feelings of frustration and tension gradually diminish. This was aptly expressed by one boy who stated, "I used to get so mad at myself that I just felt like fighting everybody. Now I don't feel that way any more."

IN TEACHING S.L.D. children, one must keep in mind that they do not perceive and retain the memory of words as configurations, the sound in the correct relationship to make up the auditory gestalt of the word, or the sequential movement pattern of letters. They may not associate sound with symbol. With this inability in mind, the teaching technique must deviate from the orthodox methods. They must consistently attack spelling through a simultaneous auditory-visual-kinesthetic approach to strengthen inner sensory associations. In order to firmly establish the language pattern in a properly formed, properly oriented, and sequential manner, the process by which this may be accomplished must be repeated again and again. Everything must be taught and over-taught. Only then can any permanently organized pattern be perceived and recorded.

Written spelling requires the automatic recall of the correct letter formation, letter connections, and the exact letter sequence in association with its correct sound and "feel." The response must be so secure that this sequential movement pattern does not take all the attention.

Since spelling and writing go hand in hand, emphasis must first be placed on practice to develop this fluency in the writing of the letters of the alphabet. This may be accomplished by using the Slingerland Adaptation of the Orton-Gillingham Multisensory Approach. Following is a description of this method.

The children should be shown each letter as it is being taught or reviewed, given the name, the sound as *heard* and *felt* in a key word, and then in isolation, the teacher listening for individual weaknesses or errors as *each* child repeats.

The children then trace a correctly formed large-sized pattern of the letter, using the first two fingers or the wrong end of a pencil and naming the letter as it is traced.

After the "feeling" of the letter form is fairly secure, the children copy it and continue tracing lightly with a relaxed hand so the whole arm motion can be felt from the shoulder, the teacher giving help with correct letter forms if needed.

The children are then taught the letter's sound. A knowledge of the teacher's correct use of sounds is essential here.[3]

When all have mastered the letter form and sound, the children should (1) name the letter as it is being formed, *h*; (2) give the key word, *house*; and (3) give the sound /h/.

---

[3] Sally B. and Ralph de S. Childs, *Sounds of English* (Cambridge, Mass.: Educators Publishing Service). Phonograph record.

Large key cards should be placed on the wall for the child's quick and easy reference when he is in doubt or before he makes a "guessing mistake."

The letters may be grouped for similar movement patterns:

Manuscript:

b f h k l t   p
a c d g o qu s e
i j m n r u   y v w x z

Cursive:

Spelling should now begin with letters as single elements of sound.

The teacher may ask: "What consonant says /h/?" One child answers: "H (forming the letter in the air as he names it), *house*, /h/." The children repeat, then write the letter on paper. Later the response may be simply, "*H*, /h/."

To further develop automatic response, say: "Make *b*," "Make *a*," "Make /f/," the children writing, naming, tracing, and making the next letter as directed. A rhythm should be kept in directing, leaving no lapses of time between directions.

Patterns should be made for tracing and practicing difficult letter connections, such as *br, os, wr,* etc. The large-spaced paper used to begin with may be reduced to smaller spaces after the children gain the "feel" of the sequential movement pattern necessary for the automatic formation of letters.

This adaptation classifies all words into three kinds for spelling. Children should become aware of these approaches to enable them to determine the method for study which gives them self-confidence.

Green-Flag Words are short vowel, purely phonetic words that can be spelled as soon as the letters and sounds of the letters required have been taught. However, unless a child speaks correctly (and this means teacher awareness, control, and direction of speech practice) even these will not be accurately phonetic for him. Unstudied Green-Flag words may be written from dictation following the pattern which is learned in the primary grades:

- Child repeats the word named by the teacher.
- Child hears and gives the vowel sound.
- Child names the vowel, forming the letter in the air as he names it.
- Child spells the word orally, writing each letter in the air as he names it.
- Child writes the word on paper. At times he retraces if needed.

Red-Flag Words are non-phonetic or irregular and must be "learned as wholes" because every sound cannot be heard. (While giving practice, the words are listed on the board accordingly as Red-Flag or Green-Flag words.) The phonetic parts should be noted and the difficult parts are underlined or stressed. In *laugh,* only the *l* is easy. The *augh* has to be learned as a whole. In *could, would,* and *should,* the beginning and ending sounds can be heard, but the *oul* must be learned, so the entire word is learned by this procedure:

- Child copies the word.
- The teacher checks for correct spelling and letter forms.
- Child traces over the letter lightly, naming each letter as it is formed.
- When he feels he has learned the word, he closes his eyes and tries writing the word in the air. He is encouraged to realize that if his hand stops, his brain is no longer directing his hand, so he hasn't learned the word and must do more tracing. He may also try writing the word and checking it with the correct pattern.

9

● The teacher may give the final checkup by dictating as words, in phrases, or as part of the dictation lesson.

Yellow-Flag Words, or ambiguous words, can be spelled in more than one way as far as the vowel or consonant sound is concerned. Spelling of these words begins after the vowel digraphs, diphthongs, and phonograms are introduced. (They will have been used for reading a considerable time before they are introduced for spelling unless given as "learned words.") From now on, spelling becomes more complicated.

Children in the third and fourth grades, having had training in this way, should acquire the ability to recall all the ways of spelling a given vowel or consonant sound that they have been taught:

/ā/	/ē/	/ī/	/ō/
a	e	i	o
a-e	e-e	i-e	o-e
ai	ee	igh	oa
ay	ea	ie	ow
eigh	ie		
ea	y	y	

/ū/	/ōō/	/ĕ/	/ou/
u		e	ou
u-e	u-e	ea	ow
ew	ew		

/c/	/au/	/ĭ/	/oi/
c	au	i	oi
k	aw	y	oy
ck			

	/ch/	/j/
er	ch	j
ir	tch	dge
ur		

PRACTICE should be given, in studying, in how to listen for or take note of the vowel sound and then to make a selection.

● Child repeats the word given by the teacher. *(Grain.)*

● Child hears and gives the vowel sound, /ā/. After working with the different ways that spell /ā/, the children will discover that /ā/ followed by a consonant sound could be *ai, a-e,* or *eigh;* that *ay* usually occurs at the end of a word or syllable, and that *ea* is found in only a few words.

● After generalizing, the child makes a selection and asks the teacher, "Is it *a-e?*" The teacher answers: "It would make the correct sound but it is not used in this word." The child thinks again and asks: "Is it *ai?*" The reply is: "Yes, in this case it is."

● Child repeats the word.

● Child spells the word, naming each letter as he writes it in the air.

In this way, the teacher serves as the dictionary while the children get the practice which precedes intelligent dictionary technique.

● Children repeat and write *grain* on paper.

● Children trace for study.

Additional related words may be given for further practice; for example, *trail, grave, snake, gray,* etc. Mixed groups of words with the vowel sound of /ā/ may be given to be worked out and placed under the correct heading (for example, *chain, tray,* etc.) either as independent seat work or as the teacher dictates for organizational practice on paper.

Words for spelling should begin with simple three-letter phonetic short vowel words, progressing in difficulty as the children gain skill; for example, *lap, cast, pack, lash, chat, grasp, branch,* etc. After the "vowel concept" of short *a* is well understood, short *i* will be another sound to open the throat. (The secret of success is in very thorough teaching and the opportunity to "over-learn" the *a,* the *i,* and then discrimination.) Then the other vowels may be included.

Continue with the following as the children are ready:
- Words with letter combinations, such as *ink, ank, ing, ong,* etc.
- Adding suffixes or endings and their meanings to words (no rules), for example, *ing, s* or *es, er, est, ed, less, ness, ly, y,* etc.
- Words where the short vowel sound is made long as in vowel-consonant-e words, such as *pan, pane, rip, ripe,* etc.
- Words containing vowel digraphs, diphthongs, and phonograms.
- Words of two or more syllables (over-emphasizing each syllable when pronouncing them). For example, *poppin, butter, fragment, lumber, fiddle, bumble, title, rifle, pavement, dictate,* etc.
- Words doubling the final *f, l, s;* words doubling the final consonant before adding an ending (l-l-l rule), and words dropping the silent *e* (which requires special teaching not included in this paper).

Phrase writing carried into sentences should begin early.
- Use phonetic words in simple phrases; for example, *grab the bat,* etc.
- Begin with a root word, carry it into phrases, and then into simple sentences. This should be dictated by the teacher. Put underlined words on the board to be copied if they haven't been taught:

Camp	camping	to *go* camping
	camps	to camp*out*
camped	camper	
	camped and camped	

I like to camp.
I like to go camping
Do you like to go camping?

- Use any non-phonetic word, repeating it in different phrasing:

Laugh
laughing at that
a laughable matter
laughed and laughed

- The teacher should ask questions to give meaning:

List
What *did* Mother do?
Listed the toys.
What *does* she do?
Lists the toys.
What is she *doing?*
Listing the toys.

- Use root words, dropping the silent *e* or doubling the final consonant, after the procedure for this more difficult spelling has been well structured.
- Write answers to questions. For a one-part question, the teacher should write: "Have you been to the zoo?" The child copies the question and writes: "Yes, I have been to the zoo."

For a two-part question, the teacher should write: "In what city do you live? In what state is it?" The child writes: "I live in Renton. Renton is in the state of Washington." Or, "I live in the city of Renton which is in the state of Washington."

Through structured dictation lessons, these children gain feeling for form, arrangement, sentence construction, continuity, and organization of thoughts which is carried over into individual creative writing. The material used should be made by the teacher and children, but with teacher-controlled guidance to insure the right words for their level of learning, organization, and overall planning.

11

After the teacher writes the story in cursive on a large sheet of paper so it can be seen about the room, the children copy it, the teacher checking before study to prevent incorrect practice. Any errors made in copying are bracketed to discourage erasing and untidy papers and to encourage the children to "stop and think" before writing.

Words that are too hard to be learned at this time are underlined. These will be written where they can be seen when the final dictation is given. (These may be used for extra work for those able to learn them, too.) The children should note the Green-Flag, Red-Flag, and Yellow-Flag words to determine the method of study.

The teacher should guide directed study in various ways:

- Special practice in writing phonetic words in and related to the story.
- Learning non-phonetic words.
- Adding suffixes and prefixes and their meanings. (Using rules.)
- Writing ambiguous words from the story and giving additional related words under correct headings as far as vowel sounds are concerned.
- Giving phrases from the story for a check.
- Playing games using ambiguous words with the teacher serving as the dictionary.
- Spelldown—requiring the correct response used for oral spelling.

When the weekly study is over, all evidences of study are removed and the teacher dictates the story sentence-by-sentence and phrase-by-phrase.

An important part of this learning is to help children hold a memory span of words within phrases. Word-by-word dictating defeats part of the purpose of writing to dictation which is to strengthen auditory recall of a group of words.

The technique described above has proved highly successful in helping children with a specific learning disability to learn to spell, thereby moving them closer to the time when they can function up to their capabilities.

REFERENCES

Bannatyne. Alex. "Spelling for the Dyslexic Child," *Word Blind Bulletin*, VI, VII (Winter 1966).

Childs, Sally B., and Ralph de S. *Sound Phonics.* Cambridge, Mass.: Educators Publishing Service, 1962.

————. *Sound Spelling.* Cambridge, Mass.: Educators Publishing Service, 1963.

Gallagher, J. Roswell. "Can't Spell Can't Read," *The Atlantic Monthly* (June 1948).

Gillingham, Anna. "The Obligation of the School to Teach Reading and Spelling — A Challenge," *The Independent School Bulletin* (April 1965).

————. "Avoiding Failure in Reading and Spelling," *The Independent School Bulletin* (November 1949).

————, and Bessie Stillman. *Remedial Training for Children with Specific Language Disability in Reading, Spelling and Penmanship.* Cambridge, Mass.: Educators Publishing Service, 1960.

Orton, June L. *A Guide to Teaching Phonics.* Winston-Salem, N.C.: Orton Reading Center.

Orton, Samuel T. *Reading, Writing, and Speech Problems in Children.* New York: W.W. Norton, 1937.

————. *"Word Blindness" in School Children and Other Papers on Strephosymbolia (Specific Language Disability — Dyslexia).* Compiled by June L. Orton. Pomfret, Conn.: The Orton Society, 1966.

Slingerland, Beth H. "Public School Programs for the Prevention of Specific Language Disability in Children," in *Educational Therapy*, I. Seattle, Wash.: Special Child Publications, 1966.

————. *Screening Tests for Identifying Children with Specific Language Disabilities, Grades 1 - 4.* Cambridge, Mass.: Educators Publishing Service, 1964.

Stuart, Marion F. *Neurophysiological Insights into Teaching.* Palo Alto, Calif.: Pacific Books, 1962.

Thompson, Lloyd S. *Reading Disability: Developmental Dyslexia.* Springfield, Ill.: Charles C. Thomas, 1966.

Wepman, Joseph M. "Dyslexia: Its Relation to Language Acquisition and Concept Formation," in *Reading Disability: Progress and Research Needs in Dyslexia.* Edited by John Money. Baltimore, Md.: John Hopkins Press, 1962.

A Form Constancy Technique for Spelling Proficiency

William W. Wulpe

OFTEN we observe how a child can "learn" a word – for example, *how* – and yet, when he sees *how*, he interprets it as an entirely new word. I have found that many dyslexic children, and those with dyslexic-like symptoms, can be helped in both spelling and reading by the use of teacher-made charts which are used in conjunction with a spelling list. These charts were conceived to help the child overcome this deficiency in form constancy and to help "anchor in" the word.

At the time that the spelling list is introduced, I first review the words with the children. I then place, at key points in the room, charts which I have previously prepared. I do not have a chart for every word. If the spelling list includes ten words, I might have four charts available. The charts vary in size according to the length of the word that is presented. However, an average size might be fourteen inches wide by thirty inches long. (See illustration.)

The chart demonstrates the goal of the technique. I attempt to show the children that, although the style of writing may vary, the word itself remains constant.

Next I hand out sheets of paper to the children. The sheets are four and

one-fourth inches wide and eleven inches long. (This is regular letter-size writing paper which has been cut in half lengthwise.)

13

The children are then instructed to write each spelling word, one word to a sheet, in as many writing forms as they can. They may use the styles shown on the charts if they wish, or they may use individual styles of their own. I encourage the children to be as creative as possible – to use long letters, short letters, slanted letters, cursive letters, manuscript letters, and so on.

This approach may supercede having the children write each word ten times – a rather conventional form of studying for spelling. By experimenting with *different* writing forms, they appear to build in a cognitive understanding as well as a perceptual understanding of the sequence of letters, both for writing and reading. In addition, contrary to what might be expected, handwriting does not deteriorate, but rather seems to improve.

For variation, the children can use colored pencils or crayons along with their black-lead pencils. A bulletin board in the classroom can be set aside for a display of the various results.

A CLASSROOM GAME can be played as an adjunct to this technique. A bulletin board is put up in the room with the following heading printed at the top: *Can You Match the Writer?* Each child is given three four-by-nine-inch tagboard cards, on the back of which he lightly writes his name.

On the front of each card the child writes or prints a word. The word is the same on each of the three cards, but the way it is represented should be different in each case. For example, on one card the word might be written in small letters, on another the letters might be slanted to the left, and on the third the word might appear in large printing.

When the children have completed their cards, the teacher collects them and selects two cards belonging to each of two students. The words on the four cards must all be the same. The four cards, two from one student and two from another, are then pinned on the bulletin board and the rest of the children try to guess which two were written by the same person.

In addition to the element of fun, the important thing is that the youngsters are building their ability to retain the sequence of the letters in the word regardless of the style in which it is written.

I have found this technique most successful, and it can be used in either a clinic or a classroom setting.

FUSION OF NEW WORDS is fun for the children because two words are "blended" into a nonsense word. For example, the teacher writes on the chalkboard: *Crash* plus *bang* = _____ . The child may write on his paper: *Crang.* Other examples might be:

Quiet plus *nice* = _____ . (*Quice* or *niet.*)
Big plus *strong* = _____ . (*Bong* or *strig.*)
Happy and *smiling* = _____ . (*Hiling* or *smappy.*)

The idea is to select two words with different initial sounds. The youngsters love this delightful game as a variation on spelling.

The Child with Learning Disabilities in a Spelling Class

Lee Crawford

———————◆———————

TODAY the literature is filled with information on "Why Bright Children Get Poor Marks," "How to Help Children Who Refuse to Succeed," and "The Astonishing Truth about Dropouts."

We find a multiplicity of names and many, many labels to describe the children discussed in such articles: perceptually handicapped, aphasic, dyslexic, minimal brain-injured, neurologically handicapped, language disorders, learning disabilities, Strauss syndrome, hyperactive, minimal cerebral disfunction, and too many others to list. The Council for Exceptional Children, the U.S. Office of Education, and the Association for Children with Learning Disabilities program for these children under the term "learning disabilities." This is the child we will talk about in this discussion of the teaching of spelling.

The teacher of a particular spelling class of typical children decided one morning that she would give a child credit for the number of letters he could get correct in spelling. She gave the child the word "coffee" and he spelled it orally to her "k-a-u-p-h-y." With many of our children, the word "coffee" comes out exactly as this child spelled it.

Regardless of the label, our children have a block in their ability to communicate appropriately—the problems develop either in the sensory modalities of sight, hearing, and touch, which bring information to us, or in the integration of sensory impressions to form concepts. The spelling teacher needs to be aware of the growth and development patterns of "normal" children. She must realize that our children's problems are multiple. They have specific problems with spelling and need the help that a teacher can give.

In the spelling class a trained teacher can spot the child whose receptive, inner, and expressive disabilities cause him serious learning problems. Once she identifies this child, she has the opportunity in the classroom to fill his experiences with success rather than failure.

Among the receptive difficulties, problems in receiving impulses from the sensory modalities, that a teacher can recognize in her children are the following:

Hyperactivity. The child is unable to sit still. He has an extremely short attention span, is distractible, reacts excessively to every stimulus, and cannot settle down after the reaction.

Visual perception difficulties. The child cannot distinguish between lines and spaces and he has difficulty recognizing or reproducing letters and words. He has trouble focusing on a chalkboard or reproducing from a chalkboard to his paper.

Auditory perception difficulties. He either does not hear the sound, does not have the ability to reproduce a sound once he has heard it, or is unable to distinguish between tones.

Body movement problems. He cannot walk or skip with both sides of the body. He has reversals of arm movements and imitative and interpretive movement. He has directionality problems and difficulty in inhibiting movement.

The inner problems of the child with learning disabilities lie in his difficulty in integrating or associating information from his sensory modalities with previous information. With his memory impairment and integration problems, he gets words and parts of words out of sequence. He has difficulty in following directions involving more than one or two parts. He does not seem to be able to understand categories. He gets the words, the letters, the values and the symbols all mixed up. He seems unable to put together what he simultaneously sees and hears. He cannot coordinate body response with visual and auditory stimuli. The spelling teacher will have to sequence the child's lessons to help meet these deficits.

An indication of expressive problems might be the child's difficulty in saying words or sounds with a group. He may be unable to say back to the teacher what she says to him. If he has a language disorder, he usually lacks words to express experiences and the teacher trains him to compensate for his inadequacies.

Once the teacher is convinced that these children do exist in her classroom, she needs to know what can be done to help them function with success in their learning experiences. Oddly enough, she will discover that not only the twenty per cent of atypical children will benefit from these suggestions, but the majority of "normal" children will reach even higher levels of functioning through these techniques. The teacher should observe the child, watch his every move, try to notice as much about his body movement, his visual perception, his language and auditory perception, and expression as possible. Perhaps she will need a simple evaluation. It is recommended that a conference with each child be written up to file for future reference and follow up.

Such an evaluation might include: "Knows the alphabet; can use the beginning consonants to recognize words (including *ch, sh, th, wh*); can use the final consonants to recognize words; recognizes compound words made up of two known words; knows long and short forms of vowels; can substitute beginning and final consonants; sees little words within larger ones; has an awareness of visual clues that aid in determining accented syllables in a word; can apply structural analysis to determine syllables in a word; can recognize words that form plurals by adding *s* or *es*, changing *f* to *v* before adding *es*, changing *y* to *i* before adding *es*; understands how words are changed by adding endings *ed, ing*; recognizes possessives; recognizes contractions and understands that the apostrophe represents one missing letter; understands homonyms; and knows that some beginning letters are silent." The teacher may repeat silly syllables to evaluate the child's memory span and have him draw a picture of himself and tell her about it.

THE FIRST STEP after the evaluation involves structuring teaching plans with specific sequences of events. These events and this "prescribed" program for learning must be of very short duration and must be paced to the individual child's attention span. The teacher must allow the child to know her expectations of him and how he is to act. As she moves from one area to another, from one lesson to the next, she must prepare the child.

The teaching technique must include the multisensory approach such as Grace Fernald developed to help children study words as whole words and in syllables. Allow the child to see, to hear, and to feel as the teacher relates each new concept. Some children learn best through auditory channels, others through visual, and still others through tactile and kinesthetic methods. So that the stronger modality may bridge the gap of the weaker, the teacher should increase learning by constantly reinforcing, expanding, and relating previous experiences to build slowly, step-by-step. Hopefully, the concepts which the teacher builds will become a permanent part of the child. It is necessary that we teach, reteach, and maintain.

Spelling should be worked on each day and the specific problems of the individual child—as well as the general problems having to do with the receptive, inner, and expressive aspects of learning—must be dealt with. Some suggestions to correlate the spelling lesson with the problems described above are as follows:

Hyperactivity. Quicken the pace of the overall spelling lesson with shorter spans of attention required for each subsequent activity. Seat the excessively hyperactive child where he will be exposed to the fewest distractions, partially away from the other children, the view from the window, or from door movement. Sometimes a partial screen improvised from a chart or table will help him concentrate for a longer period. If he is extremely disturbing to the other children and unable to focus for more than a few minutes, arrange for him to take spelling the first thing in the morning, letting him know that as he is able to listen and work for a longer time he may increase his time in spelling. Help him to feel that his minutes of participation are valid and that you consider him very important.

Visual perception. Have the child learn symbols by tracing in the air, saying the letters as he looks at them. Another way to teach spelling is with color cues. Color cue to teach the difference between lines and spaces and to make important foreground figures stand out against the background. For older students, color cue for syllabication. Select symbols from many different printed and written forms so that the child's recognition of the symbol will remain constant, even when a different type of ink, paper, or printing style is used.

Auditory perception. Begin with a tape recorder and begin very slowly. Use steady rhythmic patterns, spelling by syllables. Teach the child how to shift from pronunciation to spelling. As the child grows with the tape recorder, increase the length of sequences. Studies have shown that the tape recorder is very beneficial.

Since no two individuals or groups of children are the same, it is logical to assume that not all, either in a group or individually, should be working on the same spelling list at the same time, nor should they follow the same pattern of word study. We need to individualize spelling instruction; each child should be programmed separately. His spelling lists should include the words that best fit him and meet his individual differences. Each child's program should allow him to progress at his own rate of speed.

In some cases the teacher can record the word list for the tape recorder in advance. She can have volunteers help her do this; this saves valuable classroom time and the tape recorder frees her to give individual help where needed. Recorded word lists allow the child to drill on the words that he needs most. Phonograph records may also be used. Commercial records are available with the 123 basic phonic sounds. One advantage of phonograph records and tapes is that they give the child exactly the same sound each time.

17

Commercial illustrated wall charts designed to give the child quick mastery of the letter sounds and key words are also available to the spelling teacher. Most textbooks will provide the teacher with an abundance of material to prepare her programmed lessons. Anna Gillingham, in *Remedial Training for Children with Specific Disabilities in Reading, Spelling and Penmanship*, has prepared detailed programmed materials for teaching spelling, but, just as for any other type of teaching, these too must be individualized to meet the child's needs.

SPELLING should not be taught without word study as such: phonetic analysis, consonant sounds, variance and nonvariance, consonant blends—the initial blends, middle blends, and the final blends—consonant symbols, digraphs and speech sounds, silent consonants, vowel sounds, and dipthongs. The structural analysis of words may be attacked: identification of inflectional endings like *s*, *'s*, and *ing*; recognition of unknown words that are like known words with certain exceptions; identification of root words and inflected forms; the principles of syllabication; identification of simple prefixes and suffixes; accents; and the understanding of compound words.

In spelling we also teach children to use the dictionary. Words may be presented in either lists or in stories, again depending upon the child's needs, his ability to read, and his ability to organize.

Dr. Ernest Horn has stated that research has consistently shown that it is more efficient to study words in lists than in context. He has further stated that words studied in lists are learned more quickly, remembered longer, and transferred more readily to a new context. Our children are expected, however, to be able to do more than mere rote memory of lists of words.

Written expression is the purpose for and the real test of spelling mastery. The child should be involved in exercises using it whenever possible; this better insures the transfer of learning from spelling lists to writing. The Rinsland study on the frequency of word use indicates which words are used most frequently in writing. These are the words we should try to teach our children.

The discovery method of teaching spelling takes the child beyond passive rote memorization and involves him in the learning process. Jerome S. Bruner has said that this method is like a textbook in that it requires a dialogue between the printed word and the beholder. It is an inductive learning method that challenges the child to think about relationships in word and sentence patterns and to discover their similarities and differences. It provides an opportunity for him to use his oral and written knowledge of language to define words and fit sentences into patterns as well as to find exceptions; it then helps him to express in his own words what he has learned about patterned sets and to arrive at generalizations about language.

Spelling should include vocabulary study, programmed in accordance with two important aspects of word study—the sound-letter relationship and the frequency of use in writing. These are the multisensory study skills for learning any word, whether in the spelling program or in any other area. Vocabulary review should be integrated into every feature of the spelling program.

Anatole France, quoted in Amsel Green's *Word Clues*, has said, "The finest words in the world are only vain sounds if you cannot comprehend them." The teacher does the guidance and the child does the work. There is no one method by which all children can be taught.

Miss Ruth Cheves, of the University of Houston, has written, "It is not the material of the classroom that makes successful teaching. It is the teacher's understanding of the child's problems and application of appropriate teaching methods that develop a learning experience for the child, which is the important goal."

Teaching pupils to communicate effectively and correctly is a continuous challenge from the first grade through the twelfth.

REFERENCES

Anderson, Paul S. *Resource Materials for Teachers of Spelling.* Minneapolis: Burgess Publishing Co., 1959.

Botal, Morton, *et al. Spelling and Writing Patterns.* Chicago: Follett, 1966.

Fine, Benjamin. "Why Bright Children Get Poor Marks," *Redbook,* CXXVII (September 1966), 72 ff.

Gillingham, Anna, and Bessie W. Stillman. *Remedial Training for Children with Specific Disability in Reading, Spelling, and Penmanship.* Sixth edition. Bronxville, N.Y.: Anna Gillingham, 1960.

Holt, John. "How Young Children

Learn," *Parents Magazine,* XXXXI (September 1966), 60 ff.

Horn, Ernest. "Teaching Spelling: What Research Says to the Teacher," *NRA* (1954), p. 16.

Reading-Writing-Spelling. Curriculum Bulletin 58CBM1. Houston: Houston Independent School District, 1958.

Rinsland, Henry D. *A Basic Vocabulary of Elementary School Children.* New York: Macmillan, 1945.

Vann, Helen W. "Tailor Their Spelling Words with Tape,"*Grade Teacher,*LXXXIV (February 1967), 113 ff.

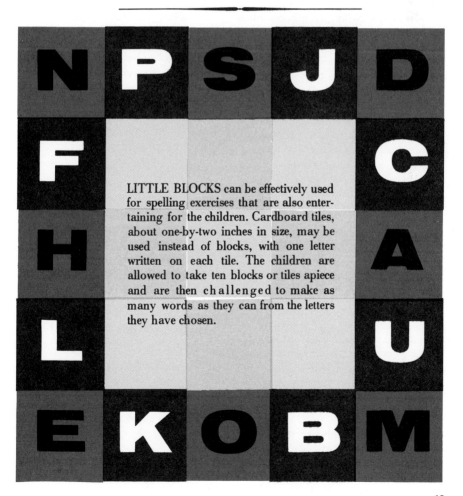

LITTLE BLOCKS can be effectively used for spelling exercises that are also entertaining for the children. Cardboard tiles, about one-by-two inches in size, may be used instead of blocks, with one letter written on each tile. The children are allowed to take ten blocks or tiles apiece and are then challenged to make as many words as they can from the letters they have chosen.

An Intermediate Step in a Total Spelling Program

Harold B. Helms

A TECHNIQUE for teaching the skills of spelling to children with dyslexic-like symptoms is one which has worked successfully with those children who, so characteristically, are able to identify all the sounds in isolation, but who cannot integrate them into a word. In a total spelling program, it might be considered an intermediate stage between mortor-perceptual-visualization training and competent, fluent spelling facility. It could be viewed as an "anchoring-in" stage. The individual learning problems of the children in the group or class will dictate the extent to which any one of the steps in this sequence should be increased in complexity or in the amount of time spent on it.

I first check to determine if the child can correctly name *and* pronounce all of the consonant sounds and blends. Using a large chart, I eliminate the vowels and, at first, I do not include *c* and *g* (because of the hard and soft sounds) and *q* and *x*. These four letters are introduced when the children have achieved facility with the basic chart. (See Illustration 1.)

When I have established the ability of the child to associate the correct name and sound to a specific symbol, I introduce other charts which depict the same

symbols, but which are written in a different style. (See Illustrations 2 and 3.)

From time to time, I find a child with almost aphasic-like symptoms, in which there is a true inability to associate on the name-sound-picture basis. Such a youngster needs an extensive amount of practice at the kinesthetic levels in which he feels the letter and says the name or the sound at the same time. This help should be given on an individual basis.

The next step is to move into graphic expression by having a "spelling test" in which I say letters in random order and the children write just the letters. This is followed by another "spelling test" in which I say just the sounds and

Illustration 1

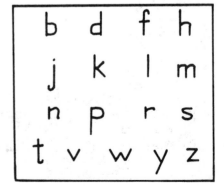

20

Illustration 2

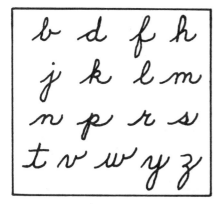

Illustration 3

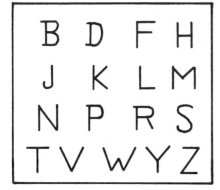

the children write the sounds. This is a key level of functioning because the child is being called upon to integrate symbolically at very basic levels. The results of these "spelling tests" should be carefully checked. Children who, for example, can do well on writing the letters but who do poorly on writing sounds will need extensive review and reinforcement.

This level is one at which I spend quite a bit of time. I play games with the children, on a small-group basis, in which I point to a letter and, for example, say: "Who can give a word that starts with this sound? Is there someone's name that begins with it?

Can you make up a word that begins with it?"

To coordinate this approach with words the children already know or which they learn easily, I introduce charts such as the following:

Illustration 4

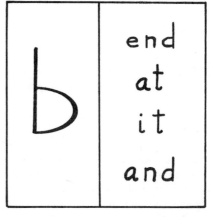

I have the children take turns in blending the initial sound with the word on the right side of the chart. For fun (and for practice as well) I occasionally use a chart which contains nonsense words. I do not find this confusing for the children. They enjoy determining which are valid words and which are not, and it eliminates the possibility of guessing instead of integrating. For example:

Illustration 5

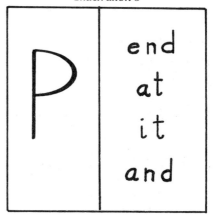

As the children begin to gain mastery of this blending, I begin administering little spelling tests based on words they have seen and used on the charts. Here again, I have found that unless the children are given supportive work in visualization and perceptual integration their spelling will be spotty and weak. Repetition and reinforcement will prove helpful.

THE NEXT device I find to be helpful is that of the rhyming word. The concept of the rhyme is often quite difficult for some children to grasp. It should be introduced at an aural-oral level. For example: "Can you think of the name of a boy in our room that rhymes with *fill?*" "Can you think of an animal that rhymes with *chair?*"

A great deal of repetition over a long period of time may be necessary to build this skill. If the youngsters have particular trouble grasping this idea,

Illustration 6

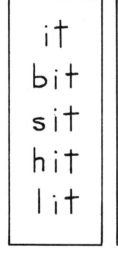
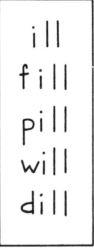

I sometimes encourage them to make up their own nonsense words to rhyme with the words I present.

When the concept at the aural-oral level is mastered, I use a set of cards such as is shown in Illustration 6. Depending upon the abilities of the children, I either give them individual cards (each set alike) or I use a large chart which we can use as a group. When we finish with the words on the chart or card, we try to add others which fit in with the rhyme scheme.

Once again, frequent short spelling tests following the presentation of such material helps the child with his associations at the sound-symbol level as well as at retentive and cognitive levels.

IT SHOULD be emphasized that the technique described above should not be considered a system within itself, nor should one attempt to squeeze it into a two-week period. Given adequate time and used as an intermediate step in a total spelling program, it is effective simply because of the difficulties dyslexic children face in generalizing at symbolic levels and because they need to build their ability to retain. Hence, earlier levels in the sequence should be reviewed frequently.

The approach is necessarily limited because it does not account for the nonphonetic elements in the language. However, because of the organizational structure, it can, if wisely used with a wide number of variations and games, instill a sense of confidence in the child who heretofore could not handle spelling with any degree of success.

"But He Spelled Them Right This Morning!"

Ruth Edgington

———◆———

WHEN discussing with parents the poor results of a spelling lesson dictated during school time, teachers often hear the protest, "But he spelled them right this morning!" Usually discussion reveals the child correctly spelled aloud the words requested. Sometimes the child did write correctly words dictated to him. Why do these apparently successful trials later prove unstable?

The answers to this question are complex, and in the case of some few children with very severe spelling disabilities, the answers are only fragmented and unsatisfactory speculations. Spelling is but one part of the expressive aspect of human behavior.

Oral spelling is a different and less involved skill than written spelling, either from self-initiation or from dictation. The latter is the more difficult. Spelling aloud requires auditory rote memory which may or may not be matched with visual recall of a given word. Some children have such poor or unstable visual discrimination and/or recall that unknown reading words are first spelled aloud in order to recognize them.

Letter spelling is a natural method of attack as soon as letter names are known. This method is effective only so long as the increasing load does not exceed the capacity of the child's auditory memory and recall. Furthermore, the success of this method may be further jeopardized if the child has visual-perceptual problems, such as hand-eye coordination, figure-ground discrimination, form constancy, position in space (directionality), and/or spatial relationships in varying degrees and combinations. Additionally, correct temporal sequence must be maintained.

Words written either from the child's own initiative or from dictation adds further complexities of kinesthetic recall. The movements for each letter needed must be remembered accurately in every aspect of direction, size, shape, and spacing. The proper use of capitals as needed, and the proper linkage of each capital and letter, if cursive writing is used, must be remembered. Temporal sequences become spatial sequences when writing is involved.

For each child with a disability in spelling, a careful analysis of errors should be made in order to discern if a pattern of errors exists. For analysis and error tabulation, use both material dictated from spelling lists and material provided by uncorrected continuous prose, such as a story he made up and not copied from a text. Some of the error patterns are listed below:

- Addition of unneeded letters (for example, *dressses*).
- Omissions of needed letters (*hom* for *home*).
- Reflections of child's mispronunciations (*pin* for *pen*).

23

- Reflections of dialectical speech patterns (*Cuber* for *Cuba*).
- Reversals of whole words (*eno* for *one*).
- Reversals of vowels (*braed* for *bread*).
- Reversals of consonant order (*lback* for *black*).
- Reversals of consonant or vowel directionality (*brithday* for *birthday*).
- Reversals of syllables (*telho* for *hotel*).
- Phonetic spelling of nonphonetic words or parts thereof (*cawt* for *caught*).
- Wrong associations of a sound with a given set of letters, such as *u* has been learned as *ou* in *you*.[1]
- "Neographisms," such as letters put in which bear no discernible relationship with the word dictated.
- Varying degrees and combinations of these or other possible patterns.

The examination of oral reading errors must be compared with spelling errors for possible relationships before interpretation and planning can be completed.

If oral reading indicates more than half of the first-grade words are incorrect, in the writer's opinion, formal spelling as a subject should be discontinued until such time as sufficient reading vocabulary is developed to begin formal spelling again. During the interim, spelling can be taught informally and incidentally through training in the development of word analysis skills and writing lessons.

As soon as cursive writing is instituted, kinesthetic reinforcement assists in stabilizing spelling-word gestalt, especially longer and nonphonetic words. Word-recognition skills as well as spelling are improved by movement patterns. Some children who cling to oral spelling, perhaps because they do not retain visual learning well, are helped by learning touch typing. For the child who has learned the correct use of phonetic skills, the bulk of the spelling words can be learned effectively, leaving the rest to be learned by sight, oral spelling, associative cues, and mnemonic devices combined with kinesthetic reinforcement.[2]

THERE are many methods and techniques for improving spelling, but time and space limit the writer to one, which is an amalgam of several approaches (Fernald, Gillingham, and others). Multisensory learning is the basis of the "Cover-Write Method" outlined below. Its steps must be carefully followed to be effective. Depending on the child's individual characteristics, age, and difficulty of words, select three to five words from spelling list errors or suitable level reading words which you wish to teach.

The chosen words should be presented on individual cards. Regardless of whether the words are written on sandpaper, with colored markers, ink, or whether manuscript or cursive writing is used, certain criteria must be applied to the product:

- Writing must be large, almost the size of chalkboard writing.
- Letter sizes must be in correct proportion.
- Spacing between letters should be of an evenness and size as to preserve the correct gestalt.

Often a small red dot to the left of the word is helpful in directing attention to the starting place.

---

[1] Samuel T. Orton, *Word-Blindness and Other Papers*, Monograph 2 (Pomfret, Conn.: The Orton Society, 1966), pp. 186–189.

[2] Wayne, Otto, and Richard A. McMenemy, *Corrective and Remedial Teaching* (Boston: Houghton Mifflin, 1966), p. 224.

The child's attention should be directed to the pronunciation, the meaning, the order of the letters, and any trouble spots if they exist. Unlined paper should be used for the work. Begin by having the child do the following:

1. Look at the word. Say the word aloud while the teacher attends closely to the pronunciation for its correctness.

2. Write the word, sounding the word as he makes the letters. He should prolong each sound unit until he has completed the letters. The sound should be clearly heard and not distorted. The auditory feedback of his own voice is a necessary part of the procedure. It is equally important that he look at the model and not at his own writing, because his vision needs to direct his hand and not just passively follow the writing. If he cannot resist looking at his writing, shield his work or cover his eyes while he is writing. This is excellent movement memory training if letter and sound matching are stable.

3. Using the model on the card, the child should compare what he has written, matching the letters in the words by pointing with his pencil. The letters should not be named, but matched visually. Letters may be sounded simultaneously if desired. All previous work should be covered as each step. Write, looking only at the model, not at previous work.

4. If the word has been correctly written, repeat Steps 2 and 3 four more times. Beyond having the letters correctly formed, evenness of handwriting is of less importance.

5. Cover all the word and the model card. Write and sound the word as in Step 2. Compare results as in Step 3.

Caution: If at any point the word written is incorrect, do not correct; simply discard the work and begin over. It is most imperative that the flow of the writing not be interrupted by erasures or corrections of any sort.

Judgment and experimentation will guide the teacher in electing to add Step 6, which is to repeat all previous five steps. If all six steps are used, ten perfectly spelled words will result. The words will not likely be lined up below each other or exactly the same size. If they are, the chances are good that the child copied from previous writing, not from the model as was directed. Considerable practice as outlined above will be needed, under direct, close supervision, before old habits are relinquished and the new routine becomes habitual.

After the chosen words have been practiced, the child should write at least one simple sentence with each word. The number of sentences for each word should not exceed five. Encourage him to vary the length, form and structure of his sentences as he progresses.

At the end of the week, dictate all the words studied during the week. If he has trouble spelling a word, have him sound it out again. If this does not help him, take another piece of paper, and place it over his writing. Ask him to sound and write his word on this paper with his eyes shut. Once he can write the word correctly with his eyes shut, it will usually convince him that the Cover-Write Method will work for him. As a result he will have more self-confidence and interest in spelling improvement.

While no one method suits every disabled speller, one of the advantages of the Cover-Write Method is its flexibility. For a child with a mild disability, the first five steps may suffice. The end-of-the-week test should show whether to continue with the five steps or to expand to include the sixth. Some older children will elect to include the sixth; others will start with all six and can later succeed with just the five.

The accompanying sentence writing can soon be seen to improve reading as well as grammatical construction. Flexibility is simple to achieve by adjusting requirements to fit individual needs.

Because children with specific learning disabilities have normal or above general intelligence, negative attitudes can be reversed by promoting interest through explanations of word derivations, semantical changes, development of multiple meanings, and changes in meanings. The teacher must, of course, be interested and informed as to the history of language changes and linguistics. The knowledge of a foreign language or languages is very helpful in adding interest to word study in reading as well as spelling.

FINISH ME

FINISH ME–START ME are two variations of the same spelling game. In "Finish Me," the teacher spells a word, giving all but the last letter. The child must then supply the last letter to complete the word. For example, the teacher might say: "*F-r-o*. How do we make the word, *from* (or *frog* or *froth*)? What letter do we add to the end— to the right side of the word?" Another example: "*S-t-o-r*. Make the word, *stork* (or *store* or *story*). What letters must be added to the end?"

A variation of the game, "Start Me," is based on the same idea, but this time the first part of the word is omitted. The teacher might say: "*E-e-p*. We want to make the word, *deep* (or *keep* or *seep*). What letter must be added to the beginning–the left side–to complete the word?"

The children might write the letters as the teacher presents them, or, as they become more skillful, they might hold the letters in their mind and supply the missing letters orally.

A spelling game such as this can be used for filling short gaps of time at the end of a class period or as a quieting activity after a stimulating noon or recess break.

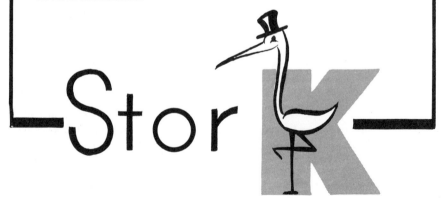

Stork

Developing Visual-Aural Competencies

Katie G. Higgins

AN INCLINATION we all seem to follow, until experience shows us otherwise, is that of initiating an active spelling program without preceding it with some foundational tasks.

When we have identified the poor speller, we should learn as much as we possibly can about him. We should find out what he *can* do as well as what he can't do.

One of the first things I do — and I have found this helpful both in terms of reading and of spelling — is to determine as well as I can the extent of his auditory abilities. I readminister his reading test, for example, but I read it to him — both the vocabulary and the comprehension sections of the test. This gives me clues regarding the auditory level of functioning of the student.

I also administer, in addition, two informal "tests" which I have designed to give me an understanding of the "spelling sense" of the student, as well as to indicate his ability to integrate a visual picture with an auditory stimulus.

The test on spelling sense, while informal and not standardized, is geared to the student's functional reading level. Following is a sample:

One word on each line is not spelled correctly. Circle the word you think is incorrectly spelled.

1.	yes	yas
2.	talk	talke
3.	knowe	know
4.	wsa	was
5.	very	vrye

An additional clue can come from such a test if you readminister it, this time pronouncing the word. For example:

On each line there are two words. One is spelled incorrectly. I will pronounce the word and you circle the spelling you think is correct.

1. Yes. Circle the word that says (or is) "yes."
2. Talk. Circle the word that says (or is) "talk."

The spelling test I use to obtain an idea of the ability of the student to match a visual picture with an auditory stimulus calls upon the student to circle the word I have pronounced, selecting it from three or four others.

On the sheet I have given you are words arranged so that two or three or four all come on one line. I am going to pronounce one word on each line. I want you to circle just the word I say.

1. park	lark	bark	hark
2. said	thing	went	leave
3. big	pig	dig	gig
4. open	ever	stop	chart

1.	walk	stop
2.	very	bring
3.	stumble	open

IF A STUDENT has scored poorly on a formal spelling test, but does well on these informal tests, this should indicate that you have skills upon which to develop a competent speller. The student has not made the transition from word knowledge to the motor act of writing the word.

If the student scores poorly on these informal evaluations, a program of association of sound to symbol will have to be developed. If such is the case, the informal observations themselves can be useful as starting points.

A solid program is built for a student only when the teacher can gather as much information as possible concerning his present level of functioning. Clues to this level are given in many subtle and gross ways.

Let us say, for example, that the student performed poorly in the two informal tests, but has been able to indicate a knowledge of the alphabet — in terms of writing it, naming the letters in random order, and naming sounds for the letters. This student, then, is ready for a series of exercises in which he is called upon to identify grossly different words in pairs. For example, many exercises such as the following, given over a long period of time, have proved to be helpful in establishing auditory-visual integration:

I will say a word that is on each line. Circle the word I say.

As the student develops proficiency with gross differences, the differences can be minimized.

The goal of the exercises given here, in brief, is that of building visual-aural associations in the child with poor spelling skill. In a clinical or special class setting, the teacher or therapist can prepare dittos in advance (similar to the examples given) and an active, ongoing file of these can be maintained for immediate use.

When working with a child with particular deficits, words may be selected from a recently administered reading test, which would allow for building of a type of graded or graduated list for that child.

The underlying idea is that we wish the child first to recognize the word, later say it, then spell it. In efficient spellers this is almost spontaneous. In inefficient spellers, this must be a delayed, step-by-step sequence.

THE GREAT mistake any teacher or therapist can make is that of rushing too quickly through any sequence of activities designed to achieve a goal. It is best to work slowly and carefully and let the changes in the student's awareness act as the guide.

When the student has indicated, by his current level of functioning, that he is ready for a formalized spelling program, then is the time to move into short spelling lessons which involve the building of retention over a period of time.

i.t.a. and Spelling: Theory and Practice

Raymond E. Laurita

Theory.

FROM the outset of the introduction of the initial teaching alphabet, most educators have been quick to agree that an alphabetic medium which utilizes a single character to represent both the visual and auditory aspects of each alphabetic component was potentially a most dramatic step forward in the search for a more perfect instrument to use with the beginning reader for the introduction of language. The direct one-to-one relationship was obviously a considerable improvement over the traditional alphabet, with its infinite variation and indirect relationships.

The principal reservation — in fact, the only one which has been voiced with persistence — was a fear of how this early exposure to language, which was visually, aurally, and kinesthetically consistent, would affect children when they were later exposed to our irregular spelling system. Typical of the doubts expressed was the comment of William B. Gillooly.

> Teaching reading via t.o. is admittedly a difficult task at best, but I believe it will still prove easier in the long run than teaching via i.t.a. when children must later transfer to t.o. with all its ambiguities. We should not be surprised to find that mastery of an irregular writing system depends on experience with an irregular and not with a regular writing system.[1]

Although discussion of this matter will undoubtedly continue for a long time to come, more and more research is produced annually which indicates that in addition to simplifying the problems associated with learning to read, i.t.a. also helps to develop significantly improved readiness for coping with the irregularities inherent in the traditional alphabet and thus also develops improved spelling abilities.

ROBERT DYKSTRA, in a two year follow-up study of the original U.S.O.E. comparative study of first-grade reading programs, concluded that when compared to conventional basal programs and language experience programs (those which Jeanne S. Chall called "meaning emphasis" programs[2]):

---

[1] "The Use of i.t.a. in Special Education," *Journal of Special Education*, I (Winter 1967), 127-134.

[2] *Learning to Read: The Great Debate* (New York: McGraw-Hill, 1967).

29

The i.t.a. programs, phonics-first programs, and various linguistic programs all produced first-grade pupils with superior word recognition abilities. Furthermore, all three programs produced significantly superior spellers after two years of instruction.[3]

Dykstra also concluded that after two years, when compared to conventional basal reading programs (the "meaning emphasis" types):

> . . . pupils whose initial instruction in reading involved the initial teaching alphabet were significantly superior in performance on the spelling test and the various silent reading and oral reading tests of word recognition.

To these conclusions can be added a personal and intimate acquaintance with a semideprived school system where i.t.a. has been used as the basal program for three years, and in remedial classes for four and one-half years. Performance in these programs indicates that rather than confusing, i.t.a. has the opposite effect in that it assists in developing understandings of the essential structural characteristics necessary for the maximum utilization of the child's potential for learning both reading and spelling.

Since it appears rather clearly established that i.t.a. does improve the child's ability to both read and spell over methods predominantly used in the past, it will perhaps be useful here to discuss a possible explanation for this improved ability as well as to present some examples of improved spelling by disabled children and a brief outline of the method followed in achieving these results through the medium of the initial teaching alphabet.

MANY of the expressions of concern voiced about the effect of i.t.a. on children's ability to spell were, and continue to be, extremely disturbing, for they indicate the widespread confusion that exists about what spelling is and how children do, in fact, learn to spell. The principal confusion centers around the simplistic belief that mastery of the writing system is somehow arrived at through repetitive experience with the manifestations of language *alone*, rather than in combination with an initial understanding of the essentials of structure. Acceptance of this belief appears to be a direct refutation of the entire idea of developmental learning.

To those who have worked closely with the child experiencing difficulty with language, it becomes obvious that before meaningful learning can occur there must be present a minimum degree of readiness in the areas of perception, association, discrimination, directionality, and memory.[4] Faulty learnings, developed prior to the attainment of a state of sufficient readiness in these areas, often constitute the principal blockage inhibiting systematic skill development.

The fact that reading (or decoding) and spelling (or encoding) involve quite different skills is often only little understood. There are many children and adults who can read extremely well but who are at the same time poor spellers. There are a smaller number who have the capacity to

---

[3] "Four Types of Primary Reading Progress: A Comparative Study," *National Elementary Principal*, XLVII (April 1968), 50-56.

[4] Raymond E. Laurita, "Phonics vs. Look-Say," *New York State Education*, XIV (March 1967), 24-25.

spell with remarkable skill but who find meaningful reading difficult. The utilization of the sensory information supplied by the various areas of the brain in developing reading and spelling skills is not a simple one-step operation. Instead, there is a complex network in operation as there is for even the simplest perceptions; the organizational and integrative processing procedures involved are still only little understood even by those who work most intimately with the varying functions of the brain.

Learning to spell is a difficult developmental process and assuming that the complex job of organizing, integrating, and cataloguing that must occur in the acquisition of thousands upon thousands of configurations, each with minute and frequently irregular variations, occurs simply or simultaneously with learning to decode, is a most naive assumption. Spelling is a developmental curriculum subject that must begin early and be continued throughout each individual's life. If this process has been developed logically without inhibition, interruption, or confusion, learning to remember and add new configurations to the existing catalogue becomes a relatively easy task. For those individuals, however, whose development has been irregular or disturbed, amassing an adequate spelling inventory is an inhibitory factor of enormous consequence in the acquisition of a well-rounded language approach.

WHY, then, should a program using i.t.a. prove to be a better program for the teaching of reading and spelling than others using the traditional alphabet? Before there can be an adequate answer, there must first be an understanding of what the developmental learning process

consists in regard to language. Jerome S. Bruner writes:

> Grasping the structure of a subject is understanding it in a way that permits many other things to be related to it meaningfully. To learn structure, in short, is to learn how things are related. [5]

Thus, for Bruner, it is only after there is an intelligent perception of the relationships between the components of structure that "massive general transfer can be achieved by appropriate learning, even to the degree that learning properly under optimum conditions leads one to 'learn how to learn' " (p. 6).

It would appear, based upon the findings of numerous researchers in diverse fields, that learning language is far more developmental than it was formerly thought to be. [6] The acquisition of reading and spelling skills requires a greater capacity for recognition, understanding, and facility with the components of language, the alphabet, than had been considered necessary.

Dolores Durkin, in a recent study of children who learned to read prior to entry into school, concluded:

> . . . interest in learning to print developed prior to, or simultaneous with, an interest in learning to read. In fact, for some early readers, ability to read seemed almost like a byproduct of ability to print and to spell. For these "paper and pencil kids," the learning sequence moved from (a) scribbling and drawing to (b) copy-

---

[5] *The Process of Education* (Cambridge, Mass.: Harvard University Press, 1966), p. 7.

[6] See, for example, the work of D. O. Hebb, Leonard Bloomfield, Charles C. Fries, Marianne Frostig, N. L. Munn, Margaret Nicholson, among others.

ing objects and letters of the alphabet, to (c) questions about spelling, to (d) ability to read.[7]

Readiness for learning to read and spell ought to include as minimum requirements, (1) the ability to recognize and identify, consistently and with facility, the letters of the alphabet, and (2) a thorough understanding of and consistent response to the left-right sequential nature of language. Prior to the development of the initial teaching alphabet it would have been difficult to add a third minimum, concerning sound association, due to the irregular nature of the traditional medium. Now, however, it is possible to add this third and perhaps most valuable learning requisite: (3) an understanding and knowledge of the relationship between the auditory symbols used in spoken language and the visual symbols used to represent these auditory symbols in the printed language.

Although it is often either forgotten or misunderstood, the written English language is a sound system. The words have meaning only if one has the ability to attach the correct sounds with the correct symbols. The presence of numerous sound irregularities doesn't alter that basic fact, and any system of instruction which does not emphasize the auditory nature of the symbols at the outset of instruction, is placing a tremendously inhibiting obstacle in the path of the orderly development of an effective and consistent decoding and encoding system for the individual.

LARGE NUMBERS, if not most, severe cases of reading disability are those who have developed an S-R [stimulus-response] approach to language which, through early and persistent conditioning, has become primarily visual in nature. The possible causes for this condition and its grave after-effects are discussed elsewhere in detail.[8] Briefly stated, it is held that the condition described is due to an initial and continued exposure to total visual configurations prior to the development of sufficient readiness. This premature exposure in turn appears to cause varying degrees of confusion, inhibiting the development of normal organizational, integrative, and memory procedures, and establishes sufficient interference to effectively stifle developmental progress. For disabled children, whose automatic response to symbols is primarily visual, learning to use any form of phonic instruction as a remedial technique is grievously inhibited because of their continued conditioned reliance upon a visual, configurational attack on both reading and spelling.

Any inhibition of the orderly development of an understanding of the essential structural characteristics of the system, especially the relationship between the sound symbol and the visual symbol, would obviously have a crippling effect on the developmental learning process. Richard Masland has written that "the essential feature in verbal behavior is the sequencing of auditory events."[9] Inability to sequence sounds properly is a consistent symptom observed in speech defective children and points to a basic difficulty in temporal organizations.

[7] *Children Who Read Early* (New York: Teacher's College Press, 1966), p. 137.

[8] Raymond E. Laurita, "A Critical Examination of the Psychology of the Whole Word Technique," *Spelling Progress Bulletin*, VI (Fall 1966), 2-6.

[9] "The Neurologic Substrata of Communicative Disorders." (Unpublished.) Cited in De Hirsch, *op. cit.*, p. xiii.

AT THE SAME time, children suffering from severe reading and spelling difficulties almost without fail manifest difficulty in the area of spatial organization. They reverse, invert, rotate — in short, are unable to develop the consistent visual imagery necessary for the growth of reading and spelling adequacy. Thus, children suffering from various forms of language disorder manifest their difficulty by evidencing both spatial and temporal disorganization.

However, Karl S. Lashley has indicated that "temporal and spatial order are nearly interchangeable and, in learning to read, the learner must develop the ability to translate a sequence of sounds seen — a sequence in space — into a sequence of sounds heard — a sequence in time."[10] It appears eminently possible then, that if at the crucial stages of learning to cope with language, extreme precautions were not taken to insure the presence of adequate maturity in the areas of visual and auditory perception, discrimination, association, direction, and memory, exposure to language could frequently result in the kind of spatial and temporal confusion observed in disabled readers and spellers. The end result could be, and frequently is, expanding confusion, mistrust by the individual in his ability to respond consistently to sensory experience, and the eventual stoppage of learning.

It is believed by this writer that this in fact may be what has happened and continues to happen to millions of individuals. Many of them never proceed past the initial stages of development and remain complete nonreaders and non-spellers. Others ma-

ture and learn to utilize context sufficiently to make meaningful reading possible, but never learn to spell adequately. A still smaller number, because of the introduction of some mediating factor outside the actual learning experience itself, such as motivation, remedial therapy, etc., learn to overcome their problems and become adequate readers and spellers. After speaking with large numbers of these individuals, however, it is obvious that the residual damage to their self-concept during this period of confusion has a marked and lasting effect.

THE FACT that many millions never overcome their early difficulties in learning to read and spell can be attested to by the existence of widespread functional illiteracy in the United States. One could even conjecture about the distinct possibility of a causal relationship between the growing manifestations of violent reactions to stressful situations, and early and continued failure in learning to cope with language. Katrina De Hirsch has written:

> The inability of speech deprived children to discharge tension and anxiety by way of words and to verbalize anger and aggression may force them to resort to action and may keep them tied to developmentally more archaic forms of coping. Lack of serviceable communicative tools hampers developing ego functions of mastery, impulse control, and ability to postpone gratification.[11]

In the attempt to explain the underlying reason for the success of i.t.a. in improving children's ability to read

---

[10] "The Problem of Serial Order in Behavior," *Cerebral Mechanisms in Behavior*, ed. L. A. Jeffress (New York: Wiley, 1954).

[11] Katrina De Hirsch, Jeanette J. Jansky, and William S. Langford, *Predicting Reading Failure* (New York: Harper and Row, 1966), p. xiv.

and spell, an interesting secondary conclusion becomes apparent concerning the possible negative effects of traditional reading and spelling methods upon many learners. It is difficult to avoid concluding that traditional procedures used for introducing reading and spelling may not be the most effective or psychologically sound for the average student, free from physical, mental, and environmental deficit. It may also be logically concluded that for those who do indeed suffer from a variety of handicaps, present teaching techniques may, in fact, be positively harmful since they assume a degree of readiness not actually present in large numbers of students.

THE REASONS then for the improved capacity of children in learning reading and spelling, when introduced to language through the medium of the initial teaching alphabet, can be found in its developmental logic and its consistency, and can be summed up as follows:

• The presence of one character to represent both the auditory and the visual aspects of each symbol reduces significantly the tendency to develop confused responses during the crucial initial exposure to language symbols and thus enhances the child's ability to make firm and lasting associations. It is the presence of considerable interference, resulting from numerous faulty associations, that greatly impedes both the developmental learning process and the remediation of all degrees of disability.

• The direct relationship which exists between the auditory and the visual representations aids the learner significantly in the development of the structural understandings essential for both reading and spelling. The more basic the understanding of basic structure, the more rapid is the development of the learner's capacity to make meaningful generalizations and thus proceed to the stage of independent learning.

• The presence of a single symbol greatly assists the development of the perceptual and discriminatory facility so necessary if the child is to be able to make maximum use of his learnings. A meaningful approach to language develops only when the learner acquires great facility with the many and diverse manifestations of language to which he is exposed daily.

• The ability of the child to respond to symbols kinesthetically has the twofold effect of allowing for the reinforcement of learnings from the outset by utilizing a variety of sensory experiences and at the same time providing the teacher with a written diagnostic record of the child's difficulties. Children who experience difficulty are immediately apparent, for understanding of the basic elements of the alphabet is essential to forward movement and any defect in understanding is immediately apparent.

• The presence of a single symbol has perhaps its greatest effect in the development of improved ability to respond to the left-right directional component in language, so essential for decoding, understanding, and encoding meaningful language structures. The reinforcing experience of a direct relationship between the auditory, visual, and kinesthetic aspects of language in responding in a consistent left-right direction greatly inhibits the development of both spatial and temporal confusion and, most importantly, assists in the rapid clarification of confusions once they have been developed in the disabled learner.

Practice.

AFTER using i.t.a. with hundreds of disabled children, among them numerous brain-injured, neurologically handicapped, sensory-defective, and culturally deprived children, it has been observed that i.t.a. assists significantly in instituting progress toward the ideal of enabling youngsters to clarify and understand the causes of their confusions. At the same time, i.t.a. presents them with a relatively simple and logical explanation of basic language structure, so that progress in the development of readiness in the basic areas of perception, association, discrimination, direction, and memory can be established. With this improved state of readiness, the development of reading and spelling skills can proceed in a more normal, logical, and sequential manner.

Children who perceive language clearly, consistently, and in the correct direction and who are able to reinforce learnings almost immediately by kinesthetic action, can be taught to both read and spell. If they are not inhibited by the presence of physical, neurological, or gross sensory defects, children can develop maturity rapidly in the necessary areas, and progress forward often occurs spontaneously and needs only good, consistent teaching to lead to substantial recovery.

Examples A, B, and C (see below) are typical of severely disabled children, without gross defect, who were able to recover from early handicaps and begin to achieve in a more acceptable manner in their traditional classrooms without excessive or continued therapy. These three children received only group teaching for two hours per week over a period of two school years. Examples D, E, and F are dyslexic children, all with borderline EEG's who have required continual remedial therapy due to the severity of their handicaps. However, even these children, with persistent understanding, support, and therapy, have begun to achieve in a more nearly acceptable manner in the traditional classroom. The case studies of these latter three examples are discussed elsewhere in detail.[12]

The methods used in the treatment of these six children, and hundreds of others over the last four years, can best be described as being a structured phono-linguistic approach, utilizing the initial teaching alphabet in making the understanding of language a more logical and consistent ideal for the confused or handicapped child. This method, developed more fully elsewhere, introduces a basic improvement over the traditional structured phonic and linguistic approaches developed by Anna Gillingham, Leonard Bloomfield, Charles C. Fries, and others.[13] This improvement is made possible by the enlargement of the alphabetic medium. The addition of elements enables the ideal of complete structure, envisioned by the pioneers in remedial therapy, to become a reality since there is only one visual symbol to represent each auditory symbol.

[12]Raymond E. Laurita, "Three Case Studies of Dyslexic Children in Which i.t.a. Was Used as the Primary Therapeutic Instrument in the Development of Reading Capability." Paper read at the Fifth International Conference on i.t.a. at Hofstra University, New York, July 1968. To be published as part of the conference proceedings.

[13]Raymond E. Laurita, "Some Observations Concerning i.t.a. as an Improved Approach to Remedial Reading Therapy." Paper read at the Fourth International Conference on i.t.a., August 1967, at McGill University, Montreal, Quebec. To be published as part of the conference proceedings.

THE INNOVATION which i.t.a. has made possible and which has been developed in my classroom, lies in the utilization of the variant forms of related vowel sounds so they can be taught simultaneously. Thus, it is possible to take full advantage, not only of the useful technique of comparing similar sounds and visual symbols as a teaching method, but also of contrasting them. It is undeniably useful to have children learn to hear and see the consistent similarity which exists in words using the same vowel sound, such as in *hat, lap, sad*, etc. However, i.t.a. enables the teacher to assist children in hearing sounds and viewing their visual representations, especially medial short vowel sounds, not only by comparative techniques, but also by contrasting them with related long vowel sounds found in such words as **hæt, mæk,** and **sæm.** Until now it has been either impossible or extremely difficult to teach the long and short sounds of the vowel simultaneously because of the great disparity in spelling. The resulting confusion usually dissipated any value that accrued from such a teaching technique.

With i.t.a., the child can be exposed to the variant forms of the vowel simultaneously and thus receive the valuable auditory, visual, and kinesthetic stimulation which flows from being exposed to language which is greatly dissimilar in its auditory aspects, but which can be recognized and encoded because of its visual and kinesthetic regularity. The device developed has been referred to as a pairing of related vowels in the most logical and structured manner possible in order to assist the learner to observe and cope with the regularity of language before being exposed to its irregularities. The vowels have been paired thus: **a-æ, e-ɛɛ, i-ie, o-œ,** **u-ɷ, ɑɾ-or, au-ou, ɔi-ɷ, eɾ-iɾ-uɾ,** and the lone symbol **ue**, because of its relatively infrequent use.

In actual practice, considerable time is spent in developing the learner's capacity to respond to the symbols **a|æ** as an initial step. Being able to hear and respond to the vowel in the medial position is crucial to further development, as it is in any synthetic system. Once this capacity is acquired and the child can respond to words using an initial consonant, a medial vowel, and a final consonant in the construction of a word, the most significant step in the development of meaningful reading and spelling skills has been learned.

The door is opened for ever increasing usages of language and in a manner which is far more in keeping with the habitual language patterns of the learner. It is possible to utilize forms and structures which are familiar to the child, taken from the idiom of his region, cultural milieu, or neighborhood. All the materials used with the child from this point on have a visual, auditory, and kinesthetic regularity, a factor not possible before. The visual and auditory contrast in even the simplest materials can be constructed to fit the ordinary language patterns of a particular child or group, even at the early stages.

IT HAS BEEN my constant observation that children respond more rapidly and with greater understanding to structures utilizing great contrast than with similar structures using comparison or less evident contrast. It is less dififcult to hear, and thus make firm associations with, the medial sound of the vowel — for instance, when the word *sat* is contrasted with sæm — than when *sat* is contrasted with either *sit* or *set.* Likewise, a sentence, such as "Pat can bæk a cæk," has greater auditory contrast and thus is more in keeping with habitual listening patterns than one utilizing a single short vowel sound, as in "Nan can fan Dan, Ann."

The materials used, the length of time which i.t.a. is used as the remedial medium, the speed at which the symbols are introduced, all become uniquely individual and can be as varied or as structured as the situation or the temperament and ability of the teacher and the student require. During this past year, after ten years of experience as a therapist and four years of work with the i.t.a. medium, it was possible to render remedial therapy to between eighty and ninety students in the first, second, and third grades — all seen on a group basis for a minimum of two hours per week — with considerable success.

Once the learner has progressed to the point where he has developed adequate readiness in the areas of association, perception, discrimination, directionality, and memory, based upon success with teacher-made materials, experience with considerable structured dictation, and creative writing, there then exists a wealth of prepared materials to be used either in the i.t.a. medium or in materials structured phonetically or linguistically in t.o.

During the course of my own experience, some students have been guided through the entire set of i.t.a. materials and then were assisted in making the transition; others have advanced approximately halfway through the i.t.a. materials before being taken through transition; others have been given remedial therapy and were given no assistance in making the transition,

and, most recently, rather large numbers of children were taught to cope with decoding and encoding by being taught only the first five paired vowel groupings, a-æ, e-ee, i-ie, o-œ, and u-ω, and then were transferred into a highly structured phono-linguistic approach after they had developed adequate understanding and facility with these five sets of paired vowel groups.

THE CONCLUSION that has been drawn after using these various operative procedures has been that variation in the synthetic approach used overall is not the key to success. Rather it is the clarifying effect which the medium of the initial teaching alphabet has upon the learner. Once basic structural understandings of language have been implanted and implemented with good teaching, the system of developmental education in almost universal use in the United States can cope more realistically with the students in its classrooms.

The solution to the problem of widespread language difficulty so prevalent in the United States, especially for those with gross learning deficit, lies in the utilization of approaches to initial instruction which assist in the development of adequate readiness for both reading and spelling. Such preparation would, in turn, provide children with a clear understanding of the basic structure of the English language upon which to superimpose the broad education so necessary for success in society. Without this readiness the child is simply not prepared to fit into the developmental system of education which has been so meticulously designed for the "average" child, but which fails to take into account the needs of the "non-average" child.

That i.t.a. offers educators a significant instrument to satisfy these needs can no longer be denied by those responsible for the decision making process in American education.

KEY TO EXAMPLES

THE SPELLING TEST used in all of the example cases was the Durrell-Sullivan Spelling Test — Form A. Following are the twenty words which were administered at each grade level.

	Grade 2	Grade 3	Grade 4	Grade 5
1.	soon	sweet	leave	clothing
2.	year	dinner	afternoon	market
3.	rest	brother	thought	weather
4.	looking	yard	wear	young
5.	along	many	pound	friend
6.	why	very	early	happened
7.	table	would	page	fixed
8.	spring	because	teeth	station
9.	upon	floor	push	explain
10.	close	wash	stairs	promise
11.	sweet	leave	clothing	machine
12.	dinner	afternoon	market	gasoline
13.	brother	thought	weather	expected
14.	yard	wear	young	disappear
15.	many	pound	friend	believe
16.	very	early	happened	encourage
17.	would	page	fixed	contained
18.	because	teeth	station	business
19.	floor	push	explain	satisfied
20.	wash	stairs	promise	faithful

The first three examples (A, B, and C) were children who were adjudged to be environmentally and culturally deprived, but who did not appear to be suffering from gross physical, neurological, or intellectual deficit.

The second three examples (D, E, and F) were dyslexic children, all with borderline EEG's. Their environmental and cultural backgrounds can be considered to range from average to superior.

Example A — Pamela

Before i.t.a. Grade 2 (June 1964)	After one year of i.t.a. Grade 2 (June 1965)	Present spelling Grade 5 (June 1968)
1. s	1. soon	1. clothing
2.	2. year	2. market
3.	3. rest	3. weather
4. L	4. looking	4. young
5. A	5. along	5. friend

6. W	6. w	6. happened
7. t	7. table	7. fixed
8. S	8. spring	8. station
9. A	9. o	9. explain
10.	10. c	10. promise
11.	11. seat	11. machine
12. d	12. dinner	12. gasoline
13. b	13. brother	13. expected
14.	14. yard	14. dissapear
15. m	15. m	15. believe
16. f	16. very	16. encurage
17. W	17. w	17. contained
18. be	18. bec	18. business
19. f	19. floor	19. satisfied
20. W	20. wash	20. faithful

No. Correct: 0/20	No. Correct: 13/20	No. Correct: 18/20
Grade Level: 0.0	Grade Level: 2.9	Grade Level: 6.6

Example B — Cheryl

Before i.t.a. Grade 2 (June 1964)	After one year of i.t.a. Grade 2 (June 1965)	Present spelling Grade 4 (June 1968)
1. senecml	1. sⱳn	1. leave
2. enelme	2. yelly	2. afternoon
3. rmelirck	3. reast	3. fought
4. Looking	4. looking	4. waer
5. lenkm	5. alway	5. pound
6. thermy	6. wᵻe	6. early
7. Tenten	7. tæbl	7. page
8. Semelemye	8. spriŋ	8. teeth
9. leaum ekmeup	9. upon	9. push
10. therte	10. clos	10. stairs
11. swony	11. shet	11. clothing
12. benne	12. dinner	12. market
13. boy	13. borther	13. weather
14. berylenmyll	14. youd	14. young
15. tumer	15. mind	15. friend
16. Tesu	16. very	16. happen
17. will	17. sould	17. fixed
18. Yurmet	18. becoues	18. staining
19. ylSheme	19. flou	19. explane
20. snene	20. woud	20. prosmoes

No. Correct: 1/20	No. Correct: 5/20	No. Correct: 14/20
Grade Level: 1.9	Grade Level: 2.3	Grade Level: 4.9

Example C — Ricky

Before i.t.a. Grade 2 (June 1965)	After one year of i.t.a. Grade 2 (June 1966)	Present spelling Grade 4 (June 1968)
1. sun	1. soone	1. leave
2.	2.	2. afternoon
3. ret	3. rest	3. thought
4. theing	4. looking	4. whear
5. alog	5. along	5. pound
6. yoie	6. wy	6. early
7. tabo	7. table	7. page
8. spreg	8. string	8. teeth
9. appon	9. uppond	9. push
10. cos	10. closd	10. stairs
11. soet	11. sweet	11. clothing
12. dinner	12. dinner	12. market
13. brother	13. brother	13. weather
14. yeord	14. yard	14. young
15. mane	15. many	15. friend
16. vare	16. avry	16. happend
17. wad	17. wode	17. fixed
18. bcos	18. becoues	18. stashoin
19. flor	19. florw	19. explan
20. wother	20. wash	20. promise
No. Correct: 2/20 Grade Level: 2.0	No. Correct: 10/20 Grade Level: 2.7	No. Correct: 16/20 Grade Level: 5.2

Example D — Peter

Peter was a tutorial student from a school fifty miles distant. He was seen in individual sessions of forty-five minutes, two times weekly.

Before i.t.a. Grade 3 (September 1965)	After one year of i.t.a. Grade 3 (June 1966)	Present spelling Grade 5 (June 1968)
1. soet	1. sewt	1. clothing
2. dirmme	2. dimer	2. markcak
3. brother	3. brother	3. weather
4. grad	4. yard	4. young
5. nae	5. many	5. fraind
6. vere	6. very	6. happened
7. cowld	7. would	7. fikst
8. likos	8. because	8. station
9. floor	9. floor	9. explan
10. wish	10. wish	10. promse
11. leve	11. leave	11. minche
12. atrnoon	12. afternoon	12. gasline
13. tate	13. thant	13. exspit
14. saken	14. wear	14. dispper

15. pond	15. poune	15. beleave
16. rle	16. arle	16. ancurch
17. page	17. paeg	17. contan
18. tvhe	18. teeh	18. bussin
19. poht	19. puh	19. satfied
20. stars	20. stras	20. fafful
No. Correct: 3/20	No. Correct: 10/20	No. Correct: 5/20
Grade Level: 2.6	Grade Level: 3.5	Grade Level: 4.8

Example E — Bryan

Bryan had received two years of remedial therapy in group. He had no additional tutorial assistance. There was no score for pre-i.t.a. comparison, since no spelling test was administered to the first-grade students in his school.

After one year of i.t.a. Grade 2 (June 1966)	After two years of i.t.a. Grade 2 (June 1967)	Present Spelling Grade 3 (June 1968)
1. soon	1. soon	1. sweet
2. yir	2. yere	2. dinner
3. rist	3. Rest	3. Brother
4. Looking	4. Looking	4. yard
5. OLog	5. long	5. meny
6. wie	6. yie	6. very
7. tabll	7. tobbul	7. would
8. sping	8. sping	8. becous
9. opon	9. opon	9. Floor
10. cost	10. klose	10. wash
11. seet	11. swet	11. leve
12. diner	12. dinner	12. afternoon
13. bruther	13. brother	13. thought
14. vrosd	14. yord	14. were
15. meny	15. many	15. pound
16. verey	16. very	16. erly
17. whed	17. wood	17. page
18. becus	18. becase	18. teeth
19. fleew	19. flor	19. push
20. wost	20. wosh	20. stiars
No. Correct: 2/20	No. Correct: 7/20	No. Correct: 14/20
Grade Level: 2.0	Grade Level: 2.4	Grade Level: 3.9

Example F — Jill

Jill repeated kindergarten and was midway into her first year in first grade when she was referred as a private student. She was bordering on an emotional breakdown at that time due to her inability to attend to the activities of the class and to learn. She was given medication to control her hyperactivity and, beginning in January of 1965, received weekly tutorial help. She also received

41

group therapy, beginning in September 1966. There was no initial spelling list for comparison, since she was not capable of spelling any words at the outset of instruction.

After one and one-half years of i.t.a. Grade 2 (June 1967)	Present Spelling Grade 3 (June 1968)
1. soon	1. sweet
2. yese	2. dier
3. reit	3. brother
4. Look	4. yard
5. uler	5. meney
6. yie	6. vase
7. tab	7. would
8. Spring	8. decus
9. upme	9. flower
10. klos	10. wach
11. seite	11. leve
12. dinre	12. aftrenoon
13. bruthe	13. fougth
14. yeto	14. where
15. meing	15. pone
16. ware	16. erely
17. wlor	17. page
18. beckis	18. tefe
19. flre	19. puch
20. wosri	20. stair
No. Correct: 2/20	No. Correct: 5/20
Grade Level: 2.0	Grade Level: 2.9

MR. VOWEL

MR. VOWEL may be played by a class or a small group. The teacher or a student writes a word on the chalkboard with one vowel omitted. For example, *what* is written *wht*. The question is then asked, "What vowel is missing and where should it go to make the word *what*?" The exercise helps build visual memory and auditory perception through active participation.

Diagnosis and Remediation of Spelling Disabilities in Elementary-School Children

Rosalyn Tauber

OBSERVATION, over a five-year period, of the performance of students who have had difficulty in mastering spelling, yet present no known neurological, physical, or emotional involvement to account for this disability, suggests that misspelling usually does not occur as an entity. Rather, the student who has a spelling disability may have difficulty in other areas, namely: reading, auditory discrimination, auditory memory, auditory blending, sequencing, handwriting, visual memory involving both copying and writing from recall.

In this group there appears to be a communality in the manner of performance—impulsivity. The haste with which the letters are written frequently precipitates errors. In some instances this has been found to be related to lack of self-discipline or self-control.

Initial Interview

Roswell-Chall Diagnostic Reading Test of Word Analysis Skills.[1]

Assesses ability to indicate the appropriate sound for single consonants, consonant blends and digraphs, short and long vowels, vowel digraphs and diphthongs, and application of the rule of silent *e* and syllabication.

Inability to verbalize the sound for the symbol seems to suggest lack of command of the visual image. The student is usually unable to associate the sound with the symbol when called upon to write it.

Gray Oral Reading Paragraphs Test.

Locates oral reading grade level.

Note type and frequency of errors; also manner in reading with attention to smoothness, grouping of words, and use of strong-weak forms.

Word-by-word reading, failure to acknowledge punctuation, and inaccurate word stress seem to coexist with the misspelling of polysyllabic words.

Lincoln Primary, Intermediate, or Diagnostic Spelling Test.

Identifies specific spelling errors. Selection of words from the list was based upon both oral reading level and grade placement.

Teaching Sessions

Auditory Discrimination Test.

Measures auditory discrimination between similar and dissimilar word pairs. Failure to identify those word pairs which are dissimilar has been found to be significant. Analyze the errors made in this group to determine (1) the pattern, (2) the place of difference in the word pairs, and (3) the similarity or difference

---

[1] For source information for this and subsequent tests, see references at the end of text.

43

in the sound frequencies which causes the word pair to be dissimilar.

Roswell-Chall Auditory Blending Test.

Ascertains ability to construct a word when given the component sounds. Poor performance here apparently is related to the inability to synthesize the sounds that make up a word. It may also be an indication of the inability to recognize sequencing. This suggests why such a word as *film* might be written as *flim* and why the second consonant is omitted in words having blends.

Writing phrases and sentences from dictation.

Copying words, phrases, and sentences.

Writing from recall after having been exposed to visual image.

Writing a short composition. Spelling here may differ markedly from that on the above items as no auditory or visual clues have been provided.

REMEDIATION should be based upon correcting and eliminating the errors most frequently made. The approach to be used should be dependent on the factors which precipitate the errors. Each working session usually provides a further diagnostic impression of the student's "modus operandi."

In spelling, as in reading, there are words which may be learned by following prescribed rules. However, for almost each rule there seems to be an exception. Memorization, therefore, does not offer a panacea.

Although some drill has been found to be helpful, its success seems to lie only in preparing the student to spell the word at a given time. A passing grade on a spelling test does not insure accuracy in written work.

Teaching spelling has suggested that training in the following areas is helpful:

• Associate the sound and the symbol. Write the symbol having been given the sound.

• Knowledge of basic word meanings and homonyms.

• Identify the second, third, etc., sound in a word; for example, b*l*ue, shu*t*.

• Syllabication. Dividing a written word into syllables and oral spelling of words, grouping the letters in such a manner as to indicate pause between syllables.

• Basic spelling rules.

• Spelling demons.

• Checking word lists and compositions, rewriting misspelled words.

Most of the material should be prepared by the teacher, geared to the specific needs of the student, and altered according to his performance. Some materials might be purchased. However, this is not always satisfactory. Editing may be necessary since these texts do not take into consideration regional differences in pronunciation.

The techniques employed in remedial teaching differ. A method used successfully by one teacher may not be successful in the hands of another teacher and may not be successful in teaching another student encountering the same problem. The specific method should be regarded as only a means by which to assist the pupil in learning and remembering and should not be made into a goal in and of itself.

REFERENCES

Gray, William S. *Gray Oral Reading Paragraphs Test* (1955 edition). Indianapolis, Ind.: Bobbs-Merrill.

Lincoln, A. L. *Lincoln Spelling Tests.* New York: Educational Records.

Roswell, Florence G., and Jeanne S. Chall. *Roswell-Chall Auditory Blending Test.* New York: Essay Press.

————. *Roswell-Chall Diagnostic Reading Test of Word Analysis Skills.* New York: Essay Press.

Wepman, Joseph M. *Auditory Discrimination Test.* Chicago: Language Research Associates.

A Sensory Approach to Spelling

Betty D. Madison

S PELLING is an important part of the total language program. Language skills are generally viewed as developing in the order of listening, speaking, reading, and writing. A person might well be able to listen, speak, and read, but unable to translate these abilities into written spelling. Acceptable spelling requires accurate integration of visual (spatial), auditory (temporal), and kinesthetic (motor) sequencing abilities.

At times, pupils need to be able to spell "service" words which have not yet been learned in the spelling program.[1]

Some of these words have regular sound-letter association, but many do not. For example, *dad* is a word with regular sound-letter association, while *once* does not have this association and must be revisualized. In addition, some words classified as "service" are beyond the pupil's current level of skill.

The following technique has been used effectively to teach service words to pupils with and without learning disabilities. It is basically a multisensory

approach, although for some children it may be strictly a visual, an auditory, or a kinesthetic approach. Just how the technique is used with the material to be learned is determined by each pupil's specific needs — his strengths and weaknesses, and the number of channels he can integrate successfully at one time. The ultimate goal is accurate integration of *all* channels for maximum learning.

The technique is implemented in this way. A test is administered to determine spelling accuracy. For younger children the Dolch Basic Sight Word List may be used.[2] In the case of older pupils, one can use words the student must know or wishes to know. Testing stops when each pupil has missed a total of ten words. These words are then written by the teacher on word-study cards.[3] These cards are three by six inches and for easy access, review, and study are stored by each pupil in his own "word-study" box. (A shoe box does nicely.)

---

[1] Service words are those words which the pupil needs for academic survival. For younger pupils, service words might be *go, run,* etc.; for older pupils, *mechanic, enough,* etc.

[2] Edward Dolch, *Basic Sight Vocabulary* (Champaign, Ill.: Garrard Press, 1953). Other basic lists can also be used in the same way.

[3] I have found it best to use cursive for pupils with learning difficulties.

45

COLOR is used to increase the stimulus value of the word. Each color is a clue for a certain kind of response. The following color cuing is helpful for recognition and recall of words to be learned for spelling: [4]

Black is used for consonants with a regular sound association. For example, in the word *dad, d* would be written in black.

Green is used for the special sound made by two consonants or two vowels in combination. For example, in the word *ship, sh* would be written in green; in the word *boy, oy* would be written in green. (Green signifies, "Hold these letters together for a special sound.")

Red is used for vowels which follow regular rules for long and short vowels. For example, in the word *sleep, ee* would be written in red; in the word *pen, e* would be written in red; in the word *go, o* would be written in red.

Blue is used for words, or at times parts or words, which do not have regular sound-letter association. For example, the word *once* would be written in blue. (Blue means, "Remember this – don't try to sound it." A word written entirely in blue is termed a "sight" word and is learned by revisualization and rote memory.)

Words to be learned are color cued and traced over with clear glue for study by the pupils who learn most readily by kinesthetic methods. The majority of pupils want their words "embossed" in this way and they enjoy doing it themselves. When tracing the words, they enjoy the feel and, for many, the raised strokes of the word enhance memory.

Each pupil uses, in a short sentence, the word he is learning to spell. This sentence is written on the back of his word-study card. The spelling word is underlined in the sentence and illustrations to increase recognition are made by the teacher or the pupil only as necessary. For example:

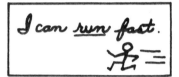

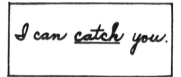

How each pupil studies his words is determined by his own best approach to learning. The kinesthetic learner says the word and traces it until he feels secure enough to reproduce it independently. Tracing is done with the index and second fingers of the writing hand. The visual learner looks at the word, notes its parts, closes his eyes to re-visualize it, and then tries to reproduce it independently. The auditory learner looks, attaches sound to the letters of a regular sound-letter association word, says it, and translates the sounds back into letters for writing the word independently. He names the letters in a "sight" word and then says the word. The pupil who learns best with a multisensory approach combines all of the above three techniques.

After the pupil is confident that he has mastered three spelling words, he is tested by the teacher, a "buddy," or by using a Language Master Card. [5]

When he demonstrates mastery of the three words he has selected, he then takes three more from his word-study box and repeats the procedure.

---

[4] Make necessary adjustments for a color-blind student.

[5] *Language Master* (Chicago, Ill.: Bell and Howell).

When first starting, the pupil is tested on all learned words once a week. As time goes by and his skills increase, testing every two weeks seems to be sufficient for sustained recall. Any misspelled words are put back into the "study" section of his box.

EACH PUPIL spends from ten to fifteen minutes a day, three days a week, working with his own service words. He studies them for spelling. He uses them in self-initiated written work. When in doubt, he identifies their sound, spelling, and meaning from teacher-made Language Master Cards. He learns to use his individual learning technique with his assigned spelling words as well.

As individual needs dictate, pupils are tested on a new section of the Basic Word List or their own personal list of words. Hence, there is always a group of words in the box on which the student is working, and a group which he has learned.

By charting his known words on a graph, he is able to see progress. This leads to increased motivation and the independent spelling study time becomes self-motivated. In turn, this leads to further independent learning – our goal for every student.

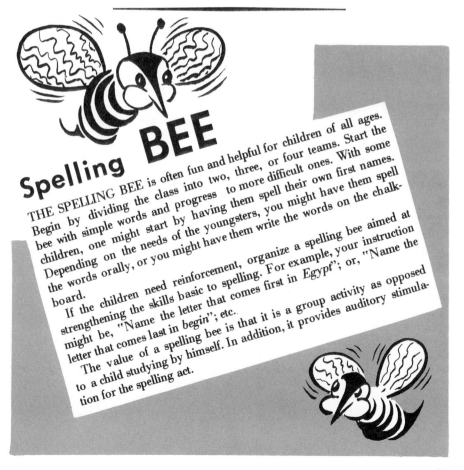

Spelling BEE

THE SPELLING BEE is often fun and helpful for children of all ages. Begin by dividing the class into two, three, or four teams. Start the bee with simple words and progress to more difficult ones. With some children, one might start by having them spell their own first names. Depending on the needs of the youngsters, you might have them spell the words orally, or you might have them write the words on the chalkboard.

If the children need reinforcement, organize a spelling bee aimed at strengthening the skills basic to spelling. For example, your instruction might be, "Name the letter that comes first in Egypt"; or, "Name the letter that comes last in begin"; etc..

The value of a spelling bee is that it is a group activity as opposed to a child studying by himself. In addition, it provides auditory stimulation for the spelling act.

A Reverse Approach to Spelling

Michael G. Powers

S PELLING is an integrative skill, and yet we so often overlook this fact when we ask children to either write or orally spell words for us. We fail to give them direct training in integration at symbolic levels. To help poor spellers, I have used the following technique very successfully and have found that it assists them in reading skills as well.

Basically and very simply the technique is for the teacher to spell a word and then have the student either write or say the word.

In initiating this technique, I spell short words, usually consisting of three or four letters, from a basic spelling or reading list. I then ask that the word be written when I tap the desk. (The tap indicates that I have finished spelling the word.) Because auditory-sequential capacities are generally poor in dyslexic children, a great deal of practice, in five or ten minute sessions, is needed before moving on. I usually dictate no more than ten words at a time. I then write the words on the chalkboard in the order dictated so that the children may correct their own papers. At these beginning stages it is not important that the children pronounce the words; the emphasis is on sequential retention.

Gradually I increase the length of the span to words of six and seven letters. When I find that students are able to "hold in" and correctly write this many letters, I return to three-letter words and change the procedure to having them respond orally instead of in writing.

When the children are ready for this shift to the oral response, I find that they do not need the slow, careful, graduated practice – from three to four to five to six letters – as they did when they were required to write the sequence. I also find that the transition of retentive ability from spelling lessons into free or creative writing experiences is a rapid one.

As with any technique, the progress of the children should be carefully observed, and they should be moved along only when they are ready.

Spelling: A Visual Skill

Homer Hendrickson

---◆---

THE following statement was made by Patricia McBroom: "The English language has never offered a very good fit (match) between its written and spoken forms. For reasons reaching into the misty past, English is burdened with such spelling vagaries as *silo, sight, psychology, cyclone, cider*—all for a single sound. Then there are *true, do, lou, brew, through, zoo,* and *shoe*. On the other hand, a single spelling stands for *cough, furlough, ought, plough,* and *thorough*. One can only sympathize with youngsters learning to read and write.[1]" It has been observed that *ghoti* spells *fish* if we use the sound of *gh* in enou*gh*, the *o* in w*o*men, and the *ti* in notion. Such inconsistent matches between what is seen and what is said and heard makes spelling chaotic. Youngsters need more than sympathy!

Developed by an Englishman, Sir James Pitman, the forty-four-letter Initial Teaching Alphabet (ITA) retains twenty-four Roman letters and adds twenty new ones, providing a separate symbol for each supposedly distinct sound in English. The result is phonetic spelling. But new alphabets adding more visual symbols, which must be discriminated by their shapes in order to know what they sound like, just add to the confusion. Eventually the child will return to the world of the twenty-six-letter English alphabet and the basic problem.

The basic problem, from an optometrical viewpoint, based on clinical experience in visual development and child development is in form discrimination and adequate visual imagery or visualization. It is not in the "listen" of the shapes. No matter how distinctly one listens, he cannot hear the difference in the symbol unless he can *visualize* that symbol.

English is a visual language, not a phonetic language. Miss McBroom's examples make clear that saying a word (to hear it) does not produce sounds which insure the auditory or visual recognition of the letters required to spell the word. With the help of six pages of fine print in *Webster's New Collegiate Dictionary* on how to pronounce words, and six pages of rules on how to spell words, one might spell one's way through her examples. But it has been my experience that good spellers do so visually, not phonetically.

What process do you, the reader, use to spell? How do you know how to spell the word which names our planet? Do you hear *all* the letters? Where does the *a* come from? Do you add it between the *e* and the *r* because of a rule you remember, or do you remember the individual speech sounds for each letter and their exact sequence? Or do you "see" the word in your mind's eye and read off the letters as you see it written or printed? Do you visualize?

---

[1] "Wuns Upon a Tiem," *Science News,* LXXXXI (February 11, 1967), 145.

Visualization is a process of visual comparison, visual recall (or memory), and visual imagery that allows one to see or experience again a previously seen or experienced object or event. It is the ability to "see" and know some thing or place, idea or concept of the past, to manipulate or view it from any angle and perspective. It is the highest order of thinking that man can do. It becomes covert and abstract, without movement; it is learned and thus trainable.

Most people believe their thinking is done in terms of mental pictures of places, events, and things and/or representative words, together with words which represent abstract ideas and concepts rather than real objects. This is visualization. The ability and skill of visualization is one of the goals toward which optometrists guide and lead their patients with optometric visual training and vision-guidance activities.

Unfortunately, because they have not learned many of the basic visual abilities, many children do not have an adequate skill of visualization. Visualization is the result of many prior experiences (movements) of the human organism *matched with what is seen* during these experiences. Some children do not match (integrate or associate) what they feel or do with what they see because they have not learned to align and maintain alignment of the eyes on what they are feeling or doing while they are doing it. Consequently they are unable to visually recall the movements they performed during the event. To quote G.N. Getman, "The look of a word and the feel of a word are both necessary for an A grade on a spelling paper."[2] Many of these same children cannot adequately motor plan; that is, they have difficulty visualizing and planning the movements required to perform a task. For example, ask a child to hop on his right foot and watch him visualize the location of his right leg and foot, watch how he plans to lift his left leg, shift his weight, and propel his body off the floor and move forward. Some visualize so inadequately that they are unable to control and integrate the muscle movements to accomplish such a relatively simple movement pattern.

THE SEQUENCE of visual development, which leads to an adequate visualization ability, has been described extensively.[3] It parallels the general development of the child through the following stages:
- General movement patterns *for* action.
- Special movement patterns *of* action.
- Eye movement patterns *to reduce* action.
- Communication patterns (speech and audition) *to replace* action.
- Visualization patterns *to substitute* for action, speech, and time.

As a foundation and prerequisite for learning to visualize, the child first learns the skill of motor control and coordination, with vision doing the monitoring, steering, and directing of the movements. The movement of the whole body and the coordination of the parts of the body, visually steered, are basic to the special movements wherein eyes direct the arm, hand, and fingers during writing, forming the shapes of individual letters which combine to produce a word being spelled. The adequate control of the movements of the eyes is learned, not only to move eyes quickly and accurately, but to cause eyes to remain fixed, immobile, on the letters and words to be seen, read, spoken, and reproduced in

---

[2]G. N. Getman, *Operational Vision*, Series 4, No. 6 (Duncan, Okla.: Optometric Extension Program, 1960), p. 29.

[3]Getman, *How to Develop Your Child's Intelligence* (Luverne, Minnesota, 1962); W. H. Henry, *Child Vision Care*, Series 10, Nos. 2-12 (Duncan, Okla.: Optometric Extension Program, 1965); Arnold L. Gesell, Frances L. Ilg, Glenna E. Bullis, and Gerald N. Getman, *Vision, Its Development in Infant and Child* (New York, 1949).

spelling. The child learns the communication skill of listening, to differentiate speech sounds, and he learns to speak, to imitate and match sounds with his own voice, to match what he hears and says with what he sees. Then he can learn to look at a word and know what it sounds like; or listen to a word and know how it looks.

Once these skills and experiences have been acquired, he is ready to learn to visualize. Vision, as a process, can then be used for the first of the three components of visualization, the skill of visual comparison. The child can learn visual comparison of size, shape, directionality, and solidity.

At the first level, the child looks directly at one object and then another for visual comparisons. In the beginning he may need to *feel* the objects to know what they *look* like. He can learn through such activities as solving jigsaw puzzles; sorting things, such as silverware or canned goods, as to size and shape; comparing chairs, tables, buildings; describing differences in trees, leaves, flowers, animals; talking about the differences and similarities of a square and a rectangle; matching labels from groceries with replacement items at the store. When he knows differences and similarities by looking, he is ready for the next phase.

The second phase of visualization development is visual memory or recall. Many experiences in preschool years lead to this skill, and structured play can enhance the ability. For example, have the child look at objects and then feel them in a bag, naming each without looking. Another amusing game which builds visual memory is to have the child briefly view objects on a table, look away, then name the objects. Removing one of the objects and having to visualize and name the removed item prepares the child for visualizing the letter missing from *them* to form *the*. As Getman says, "The visual memory of things becomes practice for the visual memory of symbols for things—words."[4]

Another exercise is to expose briefly a magazine picture containing several familiar objects and have the child name and describe them. Cut out shapes and expose briefly, asking the child to arrange his matching construction paper shapes in the same direction and relative position. Draw a shape on a chalkboard, erase, and ask the child to "make one like it." Elaborate this activity by drawing two then three or more shapes, asking for accurate reproductions. Use vertical, horizontal, and diagonal lines to form the shapes.

Getman states, "Spelling (whether the response is oral or written) is the visualization of the movements required to reproduce the letters which combine to form the word, which ability develops to the stage where the movements are sublimated to the skill level and only the word is then visualized."[5]

Visual memory for spelling can be enhanced by having the child practice the following steps:

● Repeatedly trace over (accurately, in flowing strokes) a word on a chalkboard (using large letters), saying the name of each letter as traced (seeing the shape, saying the name, hearing the name, feeling the shape while moving over the letters).

● Tracing the word without touching the chalk to the board (accurately tracing and naming the letters).

● Turning away and tracing in the air (again with accuracy of movement and naming).

● Repeating the tracing with eyes closed.

---

[4] Getman, *How to Develop Your Child's Intelligence, op. cit.*

[5] Getman, *Notes from Visual Development Seminars, 1957-1965* (Section on Child Vision Care and Guidance, Optometric Extension Program).

Ask the child if he can "see" the word in his mind while he traces in the air and when finished. If so, he is learning to visualize, to visually recall. If not, all the foundations for vision outlined above are not adequate and should be reviewed for areas which need reinforcement and movement experiences. If he can "see" the word, ask him to "read" and say the letters (spell). Can he visualize the word well enough to "see" the letters and "read" them backwards? Can he "see" the letters which are tall and extend above the others, such as *l*, *h*, *k*, etc.; those that extend below the others, such as *y*, *g*, *p*, etc.? Can he then write the word on the chalkboard or on paper?

THE THIRD component of visualization, that is, visual imagery or visual projection, is an outgrowth of visual comparison and visual memory. Visual projection is knowing the difference in the feel of objects and how they look without feeling or seeing them. It is the ability to talk about things and places without being there to look. It is what produces a "good memory," the ability to visualize past movements, experiences, things heard or read.

The development of this skill is accomplished by describing something not in immediate view (a car, building, machine, animal, etc.) and asking the child to close his eyes to "see" and guess what it is. Then have the child describe a thing for you to guess. Talk about what the things are for, how they work. Ask him to describe how he would get from one place to another—from the breakfast room to his bedroom, from school to home, from the park to the grocery store. The description should include the directions turned, objects passed and their location, color, size, distance, etc. Give him several things to do—things to get or put away, describing where, how many—to help him learn the visualization of the order and sequence of the movements in order to successfully respond.

As the child learns to visualize, he learns to look and observe. He learns to see, listen, and know more. He learns to see more in less time. He learns the visual ability of substituting symbols for experiences, and he learns symbol manipulation as a visual activity which, when adequately learned, produces a good writer, good reader, and a good speller. When he can visualize a word, he can spell it, regardless of how it sounds.

Recognizing a misspelled word becomes a process of matching the word seen with the word visualized and noting the mismatch. It is "seeing" the missing letters, the extra letters, or the letters that are misplaced.

Through the clinical experience of thousands of optometrists, the evidence is overwhelming that visualization is learned and thus trainable. Most children do not learn it well enough. If they are not given the right sort of help in learning and maintaining the ability to visualize, a constantly losing battle is fought by the teacher, the parent, and the child. If a child does not progress as he should through the stages of the development of vision and development of visualization, a complete visual performance study should be made by a professional skilled in visual care. Visual training of a much more elaborate nature than that described here may be provided. Preventive optometric care can avoid many of the scholastic (including spelling) and social problems which are certain to follow any lack of skill in eye movements, eye-hand coordination, or other visual-motor activities.

Teaching Spelling in a Splash of Color

Geraldine M. Kimmell

———◆———

THE STUDENT with a low perceptual and cognitive ability in the area of spelling, both in the oral and the written response, seems to become more highly motivated by the use of techniques presented in color. It is known that colors, or some combinations of colors do affect indiviuals in one way or another, often in a pleasant way.

In a one-to-one teaching situation, within a controlled climate, observations of a student's reaction to various methods can be effectively made and properly assessed. An evaluation of this kind can determine the real reaction or need of the individual student and can then act as a basis for perfecting specific techniques that will benefit the learner. With this approach, the following technique has been developed.

Spelling flip cards are made up as follows. Each set contains ten cards, five-by-eight inches in size. The series may consist of as many as ten sets, with the letter size of the spelling words to be learned decreasing with each set. The number of sets employed depends on the amount of reinforcement the teacher feels is needed by the student.

Colored felt-tip pens are used to make up the background design which covers the entire surface of the card. (Crayons may be used if necessary.) The complexity of the design is important. A sparsely decorated background (on which the spelling word is to be printed), with much of the card's orignial color visible, is far more distracting to the viewer than a more condensed, complicated one. Blank space is a distractive factor in that it tends to become a disconnective force in the physical act of focusing on the spelling word.

The background design may be of two or more colors, the colors overlapping one another. The directional strokes may be arc lined, circular, squiggley, linear, diagonal, or any slant that produces an attractive background.

WHEN the background design has been completed, the spelling word is printed over the design in black or any color other than those used in the background. The unusual or troublesome letters or combinations of letters (i.e., phonemes) in the word might be printed in red ink for specific impact, for example, the *e* and *i* in *vein.* (See Illustration 1.)

The size of the printed letter depends on the needs of the student and should be left to the discretion of the teacher.

Illustration 1

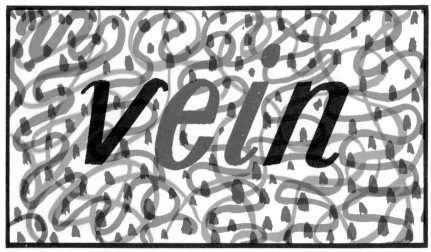

However, an important factor is to decrease the size of the letters in an ordered sequential progression from the size with which the series was begun. The space between the letters should also be diminished. For example, if the student needs primary-size letters in the first set of spelling flip cards, the initial letters should be at least one inch in height and should be spaced approximately one-fourth inch apart. The size of the letters should decrease approximately one-fourth inch from one set of cards to the next, with the spacing between the letters also decreasing proportionately.

For teachers who do not wish to create their own backgrounds on the cards, there are many alternatives available. To list a few:

- Sample wallpaper strips.
- Gift-wrapping paper (preferably with minute designs).

Illustration 2

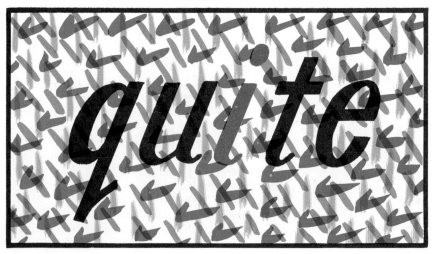

- Advertisements or scenic photographs from magazines. (Care in selection should be taken to avoid high-gloss paper, as it tends to impair vision by reflecting the light.)

The words to be used on the spelling flip cards should be determined by the needs of the student. A few suggested sources might be:

- Misspelled words from the student's compositions.

- Misspelled words from the student's spelling-test papers.

- Words from specific word-family lists.

Words containing *i-e* (*ceiling, thief.*)

- Silent *e* words (*minute*).

- Silent *h* words (*ghost*).

- Silent *k* words *(knock).*

- Silent *b* words *(comb).*

Illustration 3

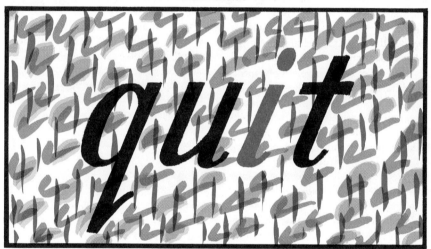

Illustration 4

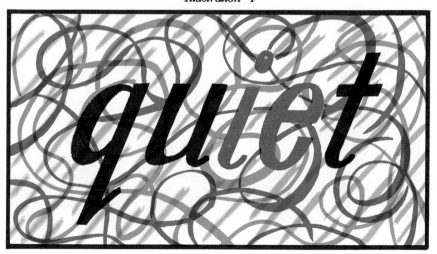

- Nonphonetic demons *(through, women, tough)*.
- Words of similar configuration *(quite, quit, quiet)*. (See Illustrations 2, 3, and 4.)

IT IS ADVISABLE to present this technique to small groups of not more than four to six children. It is important that the instructor have a clock or stop watch available for exact timing of exposure of a single word. The cards are shown to the group in advance of the actual exercise so that they will become familiar with their overall context. The teacher explains to the students how effective this type of technique can be, and particularly because it is presented in color. To encourage involvement, the children might be asked which designs are most pleasing or whether some cards, because of the color combinations of the figure and the ground, seem easier to read than others. Each child should be instructed to try to focus his attention on the center (or nearest center) letter of the word. He should also be told to try to concentrate on the shape (configuration) of the whole unity of the pattern of the word (the gestalt). The teacher should also emphasize the act of *thinking out* the sound of each letter as the child looks at it.

Although this may seem rather complicated to the children at first, they will benefit from understanding the hows and whys of the complete exercise. The visual memory concept will automatically integrate with the auditory memory input to effectively produce the correct response.

Following is the method of presentation:

- Expose for thirty seconds a word printed in primary letters on the spelling flip card, then flip it from view.
- Ask for a show of hands for an oral response.

- Ask the student to say the word before he attempts to spell it orally. Each student should make an attempt to pronounce the word even if he cannot (or thinks he cannot) spell it correctly.
- If all the children cannot then spell the word correctly, expose it for another thirty seconds. This also serves as a reinforcement for the others in the group.
- The students who are still unsuccessful in spelling the word will have another chance in the next session.
- The final step is to have the student write out the word. Do not present another spelling flip card until the foregoing steps have been completed.

When a set of primary-lettered spelling flip cards have been presented enough times so that each student seems to have mastered the words, it is time to present the next set of ten cards. This set will contain the same words, but the letter size and spacing will be reduced.

The design and color of the background of the cards should be altered with each presentation, thus challenging the child's visual system and retaining his interest. The letter size and spacing should continue to be reduced until the print size is comparable to the child's grade-level reading material.

THIS TECHNIQUE is an ongoing one. As new words that need to be mastered are detected in the students' work, new spelling flip cards should be made up. As the students become more proficient in using this technique, the teacher may wish to eliminate one or two of the progressive steps in the letter-size sequence.

An important element of any exercise is the freshness of approach that will enable the students to maintain interest during the learning-pattern integration.

An Integrational Approach to Spelling

Peter Glusker

THE SPELLING technique presented in this paper is based upon a series of postulated factors in the learning and use of language. Three primary factors are considered to underlie the spelling task. These factors are developmental in character and although they do form a progression, they are also regarded as parts of a continuously interrelating whole. A student may thus show weakness in one or more of the three areas, but he will be functioning in all three. Because of the latter point, it is important to note that the remediation technique is focused on the functioning of the whole system and does not concentrate exclusively on any one particular weak factor. This technique, however, is aimed at strengthening a primarily visual approach to spelling and language.

The three factors involved in this approach to spelling will be termed discrimination, memory, and integration. Each factor, in turn, operates in each of the perceptual modalities of interest: visual, auditory, tactual, and kinesthetic, as well as in the individual's motor function. They may also operate in any permutation or combination of any two or all of the perceptual modalities and motor function. The nature and scope of the present article is such that no further elucidation of these underlying factors and their interrelationship will be presented, except insofar as the spelling technique which follows is a partial example thereof.

This technique involves the tachistoscopic presentation of words. The underlying presuppositions, which should be noted, are that the student knows the alphabet by sight, is familiar with the elements of phonics in the words which he will encounter, and is able to write cursive. Depending on the student's skill and academic level, the words may be two, three, or more letters long, and it is suggested that each daily list of five or ten words be varied around some mean number of letters. The words used may also be advantageously selected to include particularly confusing letters or combinations of letters, such as u and n, or wh and th. Whatever variety of tachistoscopic device is used, the exposure time should be set at approximately one-hundredth of a second. Although this brief exposure period will prove difficult, particularly for students who are new to this technique, it is necessary in order to develop the desired discriminatory and memory skills. Note that the therapist's purpose in this technique is primarily to train and develop the basic skills necessary for spelling (and other language skills), and is only secondarily an effective method for teaching spelling per se.

In the initial step of this technique, the therapist presents five or ten words to be reviewed, prior to continuing to add to the student's list of words. The author has found it convenient to use words on filmstrips, presented by means of a Controlled Reader. The strip is inserted into the machine, which is set to move at a fast, but manageable pace for the student. When the first word appears, the student reads, (or recognizes) it silently. After the machine has changed to the next word, the student pronounces the first word he saw, while reading the second word. This procedure is then repeated down the list to the end of the review list.

In the second of five steps in this technique, a word is tachistoscopically presented and the student attempts to sight read the word. He may flash the word more than once, or have it flashed for him, until he is sure he "knows" what the word is. The flashes should not be any closer together, approximately, than every five to ten seconds—in order to encourage the development of visual memory. The therapist should not give any clues about the correctness or incorrectness of the student's response. Once the student is sure he knows what the word is, then it should be exposed for both the student and therapist to look at and check. If the student's response was incorrect, and he is not aware of it when the word is exposed for checking, then the therapist should indicate a brief phonetic analysis of the word, until the student realizes, as much by his own effort as possible, what his error was. This basic procedure is repeated for each of the five or ten words on the list. It is suggested that a chart be kept of the number of correct responses that the student achieves each day.

The third step in this spelling technique requires a presentation of the same list of words, either in a randomized order, or simply backward through the list. Each word is exposed in the same tachistoscopic fashion, for one-hundredth of a second, and the student is first asked to say the word and then to spell it. The therapist should stop the oral spelling at the exact point of error—the particular letter that is wrong—but he should not tell the student what his error was. The student may then attempt to determine phonetically what letter should be there, but he must also confirm this visually by flashing the word, or having it flashed for him, as many times as is needed to locate and ascertain the next correct letter in the sequence. Once the student has spelled the word correctly, orally, he is asked to repeat it until he can do so easily and rhythmically, and without hesitation. When the student can do this, he is not allowed to flash or look at the word again. All further checks on the spelling, or finding of errors, must come from his own visual and auditory memory. When the student can orally spell the word easily and without hesitation, he is then asked to write the word, silently, in cursive, on that day's list. The therapist should check the written version to make sure that there are no confusions or reversals. If there are, the student should be told that the word is not written correctly and be encouraged to find his own error—comparing his own correct oral spelling of the word with what he has written. (The therapist should be warned that this will be a particularly difficult thing for many students, especially in the beginning, but it is extremely important for the student to develop this skill.) The therapist's direct help and/or correction should be withheld until and unless the student cannot determine his own error by himself. This entire procedure, for step two of the technique, is then repeated on each of the five or ten words on the day's list. For particular students it is sometimes easier or more advantageous to reverse the order of presentation of steps one and two of the technique.

THE NEXT and fourth step of this spelling technique involves the same list of words, in addition to the list from a previous session. The student gives the therapist the list of words which he has just written. In a random order, the therapist asks the student to spell each word. Interspersed between each word that the student spells, the therapist inserts a word from a previous session's list.

The therapist spells or phonetically sounds out the word and the student must give the word. The therapist's oral spelling may vary considerably. He may give the sequence of separate phonetic sounds for each letter and thus require the student to integrate the auditory sequence into the word. He may name the letters and group them in an unusual fashion, breaking apart normal phonetic blends (for example, *gather: gat-her*). He may give the spelling by syllables, either in units of letters or merely giving the sound of the syllables. He may, and this is a particularly useful approach, simply spell the word, but with a full three to five second delay between each letter. (The therapist will find that this can be extremely difficult for some students.) Thus the current day's list of words and a previous list are reviewed. If the therapist feels that it is desirable to include more writing for a particular student, he may again ask the student to silently write either that day's list or the words from a previous list (that the therapist spells or sounds out), but only after they have been correctly orally spelled or identified by the student's visual and/or auditory memory.

In the fifth and final step of this technique, the student is asked to use each of the five or ten new words in one or more sentences. The purpose of this step is to carry the learning of the words, particularly if one or more of the words is new to the student, to a point involving correct syntactical use.

TO SUMMARIZE, this spelling technique presents a remedial approach based primarily on visual, auditory, and kinesthetic perceptual and motor discrimination, memory, and integration. Through it an attempt is made to train and strengthen each of these skills separately and in various combinations with each other. It has been found quite helpful with a number of students in clinical settings. Finally, it should be particularly emphasized that the therapist is not working primarily on building a good spelling vocabulary, although this is certainly a valuable secondary benefit (particularly if the student is capable of working with words at his appropriate grade level, without too much frustration). The central emphasis is on developing the basic skills that will enable the student to approach and develop his language functions in a more efficient and integrated fashion.

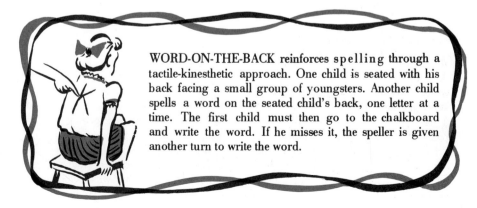

WORD-ON-THE-BACK reinforces spelling through a tactile-kinesthetic approach. One child is seated with his back facing a small group of youngsters. Another child spells a word on the seated child's back, one letter at a time. The first child must then go to the chalkboard and write the word. If he misses it, the speller is given another turn to write the word.

Nonconventional Ways of Administering and Scoring Spelling Tests

Brian Lattimore

THERE IS only one preferred spelling, although there may be alternate spellings, for every word in the English language. It is the hope of teachers that as children acquire the communication skills they will learn ways of spelling words that are acceptable in that what they try to express graphically will be understood by others.

Older or more sophisticated children who are poor spellers can understand this concept if they are shown that any spelling for a word *could* be acceptable as long as others in the society agree to it. The concept can be illustrated by secret codes, foreign languages, sign language, and so on.

The problems of the dyslexic child are such that creative approaches to helping him learn are not only important, but mandatory.

Word and Sound Knowledge.

THE FIRST STEP in a spelling program is so basic that it might be easily overlooked. Do the children know the word? Do they know what it means? Can they pronounce it correctly? I have encountered many children who had difficulty both in saying the word correctly and in knowing what it meant. Dyslexic children frequently have auditory-perceptual problems and, for example, to them *grapes* may sound like *drapes.*

When I introduce the spelling list, I have each child in the group, one by one, use the word orally in a sentence. I "dramatize" the pronunciation of the word so that all parts of the sounded word are clearly enunciated. Sometimes I introduce a "word-chain game." If the word we are studying is *went* (which is often written as *want* and *whent*), we might start a word-chain with, "Where are all the places to which Sue went?" Johnny says, "Sue went to the store." Billy says, "Sue went to the store and then went to school." Eddy says, "Sue went to the store, she went to school, and then she went to town," and so on. This oral-aural approach reinforces pronunciation and correct usage. It takes the word out of the context of something on a list that *must* be learned; it takes on meaning.

Units.

FROM time to time, it is a good idea to vary the spelling list by using a unit approach. Once again, dyslexic children often have related difficulties of a conceptual nature, so building lists in this way helps them with grouping concepts. I use for the spelling list, for example, only words pertaining to the body: *nose, ears, mouth, head, face, feet, arms, hands;* words pertaining to the home: *bed, stove, rug, door, window, kitchen;* or words pertaining to school: *desk, pencil, paper, lunch, recess, pupil, room, yard,* and so on.

The children like this approach because, first, they are involved in the selection of the words and, second, the words have direct application in their own lives. They, therefore, learn them more quickly and retain them more easily.

Principles.

IT SEEMS that "good" spellers eventually abstract their own spelling generalizations at the symbolic level. Dyslexic children need help and practice in acquiring this skill.

After the children acquire an understanding that words can be grouped around one thought, as described above, they can be moved into tackling lists of words which are based on certain principles. For example, a spelling list might emphasize the short *a* sound and include words such as *had, sat, bad, mat, lad, rag.*

At the time of the terminal spelling test, I usually add "mystery" words to the list – words that the children have not previously studied. With a list that stresses the short *a* such as is suggested above, the "mystery" words might be, for example, *sad* and *bag.* If I am teaching the initial *b* sound, I might have as the spelling list: *bat, band, buy, bear, but, base.* On the final test I would add, as the two "mystery" words, *bed* and *bend.* I might possibly add two additonal words which rhyme with words on the list, such as *tear* and *hand.* The children, of course, know in advance that there will be new words introduced on the final test and they also know that

correctly spelled "mystery" words earn extra points.

Variations in approach of this type assure the teacher that principles are being integrated and they also add an element of fun for the child.

Scoring Papers.

I once had a twelve-year-old girl who had made considerable gains in her spelling, even though she continued to misspell a majority of words at the end of the year. Had I graded her on "words correct," her spelling grade would have remained low. At the beginning of the year she spelled, for example, the word *paper* as *depest* and *dedre.* At mid-year she was writing the word as *pepar* - still not correct, to be sure, but certainly more nearly approaching accuracy than were her original responses. Grading her response as incorrect, it seemed, would not reflect her progress.

This little girl led me to explore a different way of scoring tests which I have used from time to time when it seemed appropriate. I give one point for each letter written in its correct sequence. For example, the spelling list would be set up as follows:

1.	lunch	5 points
2.	class	5 points
3.	paper	5 points
4.	pencil	6 points
5.	desk	4 points

If, at the time of the spelling test, the child wrote the words as follows, she received the indicated points:

1. lnuch   3 points
(Three letters in correct sequence.)
2. calss   3 points
3. papper   5 minus 1 = 4 points
(For adding an extra letter.)
4. phencli   4 minus 1 = 3 points
5. desk   4 points

Total 17 points out of a possible 25 points.

The children can graph their own points or, if they are advanced enough, they can determine and graph the percentages. Eventually, as the children become more proficient and the concept of sequencing is integrated, they should be graduated to a regular scoring system whereby the word must be spelled accurately if any credit is to be given.

Another system of scoring that I, as well as many other teachers, have used is to have the children exchange papers for purposes of scoring. While children can accidentally miss their own errors, they can usually spot those made by others. When using this system, I have the children fold down the part of the paper on which the name is written. I then collect the papers and pass them to different children. An argument against this method is that the child is again being exposed to an incorrect spelling. This can, however, be counteracted by having the word written correctly on the chalkboard and having the student write the word correctly next to the misspelled version.

Jumbled Letters.

IN CASES where retention is a severe problem and the teacher is attempting to strengthen this area, the following approach seems to work well. Once again, this method is to be used as a starting point for more formal approaches.

If the spelling list for the week includes the words *lunch, class, paper,*

pencil, and *desk,* following is an example of the spelling test the children might be given:

Name _____
Date _____

1. cunlh   *l _ _ _ h*
2. lssac   *c _ _ _ s*
3. ppare   *p _ _ _ r*
4. cilepn   *p _ _ _ _ l*
5. kesd   *d _ _ k*

I then say to the children, "I have mixed up the letters in each of your spelling words but, as a clue, I have written the first and the last letter. The first word is *lunch.* Write *lunch* on line number one. Use only the letters that are given. Ready? Word number two is *class.* I have written the first and last letters," etc.

Watch the children carefully and try eliminating the last letter, giving them only the first. If the words are too mixed up, instead of *cunlh* for *lunch,* try *lucnh.*

THESE approaches have been helpful for the students with whom I have worked. By starting with the errors the child is making and using that as a starting point, a student with extremely poor spelling skills is helped in overcoming his own individual deficiencies.

The techniques are not ends unto themselves, but are ways of coping with immediate problems in the process of academic remediation.

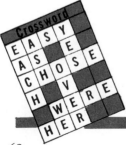

CROSSWORD PUZZLES, teacher- or student-made, are always excellent exercises in spelling. The opportunity they afford for writing the words vertically as well as horizontally is also helpful. Children can take turns at presenting the "crossword puzzle of the week"; or several children can work together in making up puzzles for the entire class.

What Is Meant by a Linguistic
Approach to Reading and Spelling?

Bickley F. Simpson

A TEAM of specialists in the greater Boston community are sharing their observations about children with average to superior intellects and no personality disorders, who fail to learn to read and spell. Each team member has found something that works with an individual child in trouble. Each is wise enough to know there is no perfect method or all-encompassing technique to help every difficulty. Each is flexible and skilled enough to look beneath the names of deHirsch, Kephart, Frostig, and Gillingham to find basic principles for language therapy.

These basic principles are being upheld by the recent insights of Richard Held in psychology, of Daniel I. Slobin in linguistics, and H.W. Magoun in neurophysiology, to mention only a few. They must now be applied and evaluated in the public and independent schools. Language disorders in children possibly can be predicted. If so, early identification and diagnostic teaching can prevent some children from failing in school.

The first principle is a systematic progression of language skills. The phonemic-graphemic code must be broken into micro-units so the program can start at the point of the child's confusion. With closely controlled graduations, he progresses at his own pace, motivated by immediate and successful responses.[1] He must not become bored by the programming or drill; however, he must have practice in automatizing the sound-symbol relationships in reading and spelling.

The second principle is a multisensory approach to language. Listening, speaking, reading, spelling, handwriting, and composition are taught as one unit so that reinforcement by the aural, oral, visual, tactile, and kinesthetic pathways to the brain can take place. A perceptual-motor profile on each child must be assessed by the teacher in order that the strong modality can be used for teaching. Training which strengthens the weak modality must relate in some way to the core language program.

The third principle is a spiral curriculum which revisits the basic concepts of sentence, noun, verb, theme, and metaphor until the formal terminology of grammar and literature is learned.[2] These concepts must be accurate, as negative learning only adds to the child's confusion.

The fourth principle is an inductive approach to generalizations about language. The child must be led to discover the basic rules and modifications for himself so he can transfer them effectively to new situations.

---

[1] N. Dale Bryant, "Some Principles of Remedial Instruction for Dyslexia," *The Reading Teacher* (April 1965).

[2] Jerome S. Bruner, *The Process of Education* (Cambridge, Mass.: Harvard University Press, 1961).

The fifth and most important principle is an emphasis on the pattern and structure of language, on the fact that English is not as illogical as it might appear. This is what is meant by a "linguistic" approach to reading and spelling. A child with coding problems needs a different type of educational therapy from that of a child with conceptual problems. His automatization, sequencing, and organization skills have to be strengthened by learning to break the code in reading, to apply rules and modifications in spelling, and to substitute and expand sentence patterns in writing.

Goals in any training program for language therapists are three-fold: sensitivity and skill in order to identify and describe potential language disability in children; leadership in multidisciplinary sessions in order to prescribe the educational program; and background and flexibility in order to judge materials, techniques, and machines as claims are made about them.

What guidelines are there for present corrective programs? Children with coding difficulties must be shown how to structure isolated sounds and symbols for immediate pattern recognition and to generalize rules for the correspondence between sounds and symbols. Thus, a "linguistic" program is defined as one in which the sounds are *accurately* placed in visual patterns (CVC, CVCe, CVVC, CV) and regularized by structure according to the frequency of the pattern. Once the regular pattern is grasped, the child learns to modify the rule. He must also learn that a certain percentage of the words are irregular. Gattegno regularizes spelling by the use of color; Pitman and Fry by the addition of visual symbols. These programs, thus, cannot be called "linguistic," according to the preceding definition.

THE LABEL "linguistic" is not the miracle program some reading experts would lead you to believe. (A course in applied linguistics, however, *is* essential for language therapists.) The competency of the teacher is the critical factor. So is the enthusiasm of the child for the materials. We would like to list additional factors that must be present in a "perfect" reading and spelling system.

There should be progression of a reasonable story in sentences from the beginning of the program, not merely the introduction of isolated sounds and/or letters. A literary quality to the reading must evolve as quickly as possible.[3] Spelling generalizations must be accurately presented and ordered in proportionate importance as the child learns to break the code.

If confusion occurs, emphasis on motor and/or eye dominance training characteristic of the programs of Ray H. Barsch and G.N. Getman can be beneficial to many children. So can the programs of Robert Russell and Ruth Cheves, but they must always be prescribed in relation to the development of alphabet skills and with regard to the perceptual-motor profile of the individual child.

The critical issue of any spelling program centers around "the set of diversity." It would appear from the research finding of Project Literacy[4] that potential generalizations are derived from a differentiation approach rather than a simple sequence method.

A simple sequence method begins with one syllabic pattern (CVC) as in the *Merrill Linguistic Readers* and the *Structural Reading Series* or (CVCe) as in *The*

---

[3] See for example, Ann Hughes (ed.), *Open Court Basic Readers* (LaSalle, Ill.: Open Court Publishing Co., 1965).

[4] Joanna P. Williams, "Project Literacy," *The New England Reading Association Journal*, II (Winter 1967).

Phonovisual Method,[5] and progresses slowly or rapidly, depending on the series, through the remaining regular patterns. A slow, minutely programmed method, heavy with drill, is characteristic of the Bloomfield, Sullivan, and Woolman materials.[6] Programs that move swiftly through the difficult short vowels, particularly short *a* and *e*, are the SRA, Harper and Row, and Lippincott texts.[7]

A differentiation approach would secure one short vowel pattern (CaC), then contrast it with the long vowel pattern (CaCe). Rather than to continue through the regular short vowels (CiC, CuC, CeC, CoC), modifications to the general rule would be introduced immediately, such as the sound of *a* followed by *y*, *w*, or *r*. It is a conjecture by some psychologists that the problem of transferring rules to irregular situations (when *ea* does not say *meat,* but *head, great,* or *create*) would be eased by this method.

There are still many words—nearly ten per cent—that resist linguistic analysis. Content words, such as *one* and *pretty,* have to be burned in with contextual clues, flashcards, and kinesthetic tracing. Function words, such as *was* and *from,* must have the additional reinforcement of syntactical analysis. It is this area of generative grammar, perhaps, that linguistics will make its most important contribution to language therapy.

---

[5] Charles C. Fries, Rosemary Wilson, and Mildred K. Rudolph, *Merrill Linguistic Readers* (Columbus, Ohio: Charles E. Merrill, 1965); Cathering Stern, *Structural Reading Series* (Syracuse, N.Y.: L. W. Singer, 1966); Lucille Schoolfield and Josephine Timberlake, *The Phonovisual Method* (Washington, D.C.: Phonovisual Products).

[6] Leonard Bloomfield and Clarence L. Barnhart, *Let's Read* (Detroit, Mich.: Wayne State University Press, 1961); Maurice

William Sullivan, *Behavioral Research Laboratories' Reading Program* (Palo Alto, Calif.: Ladera Professional Center, 1966).

[7] Donald Rasmussen and Lynn Goldberg, *Basic Reading Series: A Pig Can Jig* (Chicago, Ill.: Science Research Associates, 1964); Henry Lee Smith and Clara Stratemeyer, *The Linguistic Science Readers* (Evanston, Ill.: Harper and Row, 1963); Glenn McCracken and Charles Walcutt, *Basic Reading Series* (New York: Lippincott, 1963–65).

REFERENCES

Barsch, Ray H. *A Movigenic Curriculum Guide.* Bulletin No. 25. Madison Wisc.: Bureau for Handicapped Children, 1965.

Cheves, Ruth. *Visual-Motor Perception Teaching Materials.* Boston, Mass.: Teaching Resources, Inc., 1965.

Chomsky, Noam. *Syntactic Structures.* Gravenhage (The Hague): Mouton, 1962.

De Hirsch, Katrina, Jeanette Jansky, and William S. Langford. *Predicting Language Failure.* New York: Harper and Row, 1966.

Fernald, Grace M. *Remedial Techniques in Basic School Subjects.* New York: McGraw-Hill, 1943.

Frostig, Marianne, and David Horne. *The Frostig Program for the Development of Visual Perception.* Chicago, Ill.: Follett, 1964.

Getman, G. N., and E. R. Kane. *The Physiology of Readiness.* Minneapolis, Minn.: Programs to Accelerate School Success, 1964.

Gillingham, Anna, and Bessie W. Stillman. *A Linguistic Analysis of Remedial Training for Children with Specific Disability in Reading, Spelling, and Penmanship.*

Cambridge, Mass.: Educators Publishing Service, 1960.

Held, Richard, and Jerold Rekosh. "Motor Sensory Feedback and the Geometry of Visual Space," *Science,* CXXXXI (August 23, 1963).

Hodges, R. E., and E. Hugh Rudolph. "Searching Linguistics for Clues for the Teaching of Spelling," *Elementary English* (May 1965).

Kephart, Newell C. *The Slow Learner in the Classroom.* Columbus, Ohio: Charles E. Merrill, 1960.

Magoun, H. W. *The Waking Brain.* Springfield, Ill.: Charles C. Thomas, 1963.

Roberts, Paul. *Roberts English Series.* New York: Harcourt, Brace and World, 1966.

Russell, Robert. *A Program of Special Classes for Children with Learning Disability.* East Orange, N.J.: New Jersey Association for B.I.C., 1965.

Slobin, Daniel I. "Imitation and the Acquisition of Syntax." Paper presented at the Second Research Planning Conference for Project Literacy, Chicago, Illinois, August 7, 1964.

Memory for Design, Shapes, and Forms

Robert K. Bruce

POOR SPELLERS have many kinds of related dysfunctions. A typical pattern is that in which all the letters of the word are present but are misplaced. *Girl* becomes *gril, felt* becomes *left, tub* becomes *but,* and so on.

The approach described in this article has proved successful for helping intellectually capable children who are having difficulties in the language areas.

In the first phase of this approach, the children are requested to retain and then draw designs which are placed before them on individual cards. Accuracy of duplication is important, but size is not. In fact requiring the child to reduce the size of the design is an important ingredient in the technique.

For example, each child in a small group is given a set of six numbered cards. Each card, a five-inch square of tagboard, has a single design on one side and is blank on the reverse side. (Illustration I.) Each child also

Illustration I

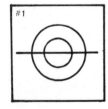
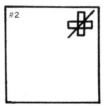

is given a dittoed copy sheet with six numbered spaces marked off, one for each design. (Illustration II.)

Illustration II

NAME	
DATE	
#1	#2
#3	#4
#5	#6

The children are given the following instructions:

You each have a set of six cards. There is a design on each card. You also have a sheet of paper with numbered spaces on it. I want you to look at each design carefully. When you think you can remember it perfectly, turn it over and then draw it from memory in the correct space. Remember, you can't look at it again after you have turned it over.

In the early stages, you may want to allow the children who are having difficulty the opportunity to take "one more look."

The design cards should be so structured that a different color is used on each card. For example, Card No. 1 may have a green design, the design on Card No. 2 may be in red, and so on. The children are requested to draw their design in the same color as the original.

It is a good idea to have up to six different sets of these cards available. It is also important to review the work of the children as soon as possible following the rendering of their representations. If it is obvious that a child is continuing to have difficulty, he should be changed over to similar activities which involve direct copying.

Direct copying, when necessary, should start with two figures to a card. (See Illustration III.) The children who were poor on the retention should be "promoted" to more involved designs, but the design card should always be kept face up in front of them. As they gain proficiency in duplicating the design, see if they can reproduce it when the master card is slightly turned or angled to the left or the right. The transition to retention may prove difficult, so it should be handled slowly and carefully.

Illustration III

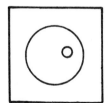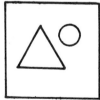

AS THE CHILDREN become proficient and are achieving greater speed and accuracy, they are ready to move to the next level of complexity. This level involves the use of

sequenced pattern c a r d s. (Illustration IV.)

Illustration IV

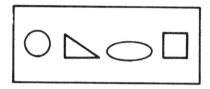

Again, each child is given six numbered cards and a form on which to draw his representation. He is again allowed to look at the card for as long as he wishes, but he may not look at it again after he has turned it over.

At first the child is called upon to retain a sequence of different shapes, all in the same color. As he advances, different colors are used in the same sequence. For example, initially, all the forms on one card might be blue. At a later time, the circle on the card might be red, the triangle orange, the oval green, and the square brown. The child is now required to retain the shapes, their sequence, and the correct colors.

Throughout this procedure, the teacher should remember that if a child is having extreme difficulty retaining the forms or sequences, he should be returned to direct copying of simple forms or he should be given the allowance of "extra looks" at the design.

A variation of this approach may be used when one therapist is working with one youngster. A simple design may be drawn on the chalkboard and the child is allowed to look at it for as long as he wishes. When he indicates he is ready, the therapist erases the design and the child draws it from memory on a sheet of paper. This paper is then set aside.

Next, the therapist draws the same design on the chalkboard, but adds a new design element to it. Once again the child looks at the design until he feels he has retained it, the therapist erases it from the chalkboard, and on another piece of paper the child draws it as an entirely new design. This process may continue up to four or five times, with additions each time. It depends, however, on how well the child retains the old portions and how complex the design becomes. (The therapist, of course, should have a master copy from which the original design and the expanded versions are drawn.)

A gradual transition away from geometric forms is made by the teacher. She begins instead to present forms in which the same figure is used, but in various spatial rotations. (Illustration V.)

Illustration V

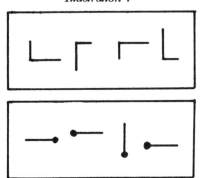

T HE FINAL STAGE in this approach to developing retention is to move the child into the retention of sentences. Again, the youngster is allowed to look at the sentence to be replicated for as long as he wishes, but once he flips the card he should not be permitted to look at it again. The sentences presented to the child may or may not include words known to him. The teacher should try both methods, keeping in mind always that the goal *at this point* is the building of retention.

This method may also be used to develop auditory retention. The teacher might dictate a sequence such as: *9 - G - H - 7 - Y.* The child is then asked to repeat it. Sequences of differing lengths may be given, or sequences of letters only or numbers only. A record should be kept of the point at which the child loses the sequence or where he begins to lose or substitute items.

When the child is proficient at repeating the sequences orally, he should be asked to write them. The final element of complexity in the aural training is to delay the graphic response by three seconds. For example, the teacher may say, "9 - G - H - 7 - Y." The child must wait three seconds and then write the sequence. Children who perform well without the delay may have extreme difficulty when asked to "hold in" the sequence. This momentary storing of the sequence, brief as it may be, is equivalent to the turning of the card in the visual approach to retention. It is the "test." If the child is able to do this, he will be ready for a concentrated program in holding in words from a spelling list.

Training of the type described in this article must be extended over a considerable period of time. The progress of the child should be watched carefully before moving on to more complex states. As necessary, the child should be given ample time for review and reinforcement. The teacher should also watch the child's total language program for all signs of integration and diffusion. If the technique has been effective, its results will be noticeable in all areas.

Developmental Teaching
for Remedial Spelling

Ellwood C. Lilly

Sarah A. Shafer

IN 1938 Temple Fay hypothesized that the growth and development of the central nervous system follows the pattern of its origin over time. He pointed out the similarity between the wrigglings and crawlings of the first amphibians and those of the infant in his early efforts to move about. According to Fay, function precedes structure. What is used grows and, if its growth has survival value for the species, it is passed on to future generations. Those without the necessary refinement in structure tend not to survive long enough to procreate.

Muscle tissue needs a blood supply. As muscle tissue receives more blood, it does more growing and it draws to it the neurilemmal sheath through which the axons of neurons find their way to the muscle and gain control over its contractions and relaxations. This is structure and function, and the function is exercise.

As each individual within a species develops, many factors can intervene to cause variations in the developmental sequence. Some of these may be genetic, some nutritional, some pathological, some lethal to the organism, but most are probably only sufficient to make each individual an individual and to be responsible for differences in behavior.

Among such differences are variations in learning ability which may range from a generalized difficulty in learning to specific areas of disability.

Among such specific disabilities may be found such things as developmental dyslexia, acalculia, and spelling problems. In computer terms, reading, arithmetic, and spelling may be considered to represent the "soft goods" while the neurological systems which must process them represent the "hard goods."

It is our contention that it is difficult, if not impossible, to process "soft goods" when the "hard goods" are inadequate or in poor repair. Therefore, we teach a series of exercises based on a developmental sequence of motor patterns and oriented toward the growth and organization of the "hard goods" so that the "soft goods" may be efficiently utilized.

This series of exercises includes the following steps:

Patterning in Place. This is a homolateral exercise done lying on the stomach with the arm and leg on the same side flexed and the head turned toward the flexed arm. This position is reversed going from right to left and back to right and so on.

Crawling. This follows patterning in place and makes use of the same homolateral pattern except that the feet and arms are now used to propel the body across the floor. During this phase, biaural and biocular growth are encouraged since this position makes possible only the alternate use of the ipsilateral eye and ear. Thus the eyes and the ears are given opportunity for equal growth and development.

Creeping. This is done on the hands and knees in a diagonal pattern, which facilitates emergence of binocular and binaural growth since eyes and ears are now used simultaneously rather than alternately. This is the period of development of image fusion without which reading and spelling are difficult. In the creeping position, the head is turned toward the lead hand and the child is instructed to focus on that hand. In that position, the hand tends to be a reading distance from the eyes and the position of the head makes it impossible for the "looking" to be done with one eye only. Thus proper use and development of both eyes is encouraged.

Diagonal walking. In the walking position, the use of steropic vision and stereophonic hearing is encouraged.

Dominance Training. At this stage, the emphasis is on teaching the use of the eye, ear, hand, and foot of the preferred side to act as leaders in both skilled and unskilled activities.

While the subject of laterality is far too complex and still too controversial to be discussed at length in this article, it would appear that efficiency (which is not lacking in nature) would dictate the use of one of the two cerebral hemispheres for the establishment of neural centers related to those strictly human functions of thought, speech, writing, reading, and spelling. To date, no way of accomplishing this, other than by using the feedback from peripheral activity, has been discovered.

While we are aware that many individuals who function extremely well at the intellectual level are not blessed with one-sided cerebral organization, we postulate that there is no evidence to indicate how much better even their functioning might be were they better cerebrally organized. Therefore, we teach the child to develop one-sided dominance.

A program of visual pursuit exercises is also carried on in order to teach the child to use both eyes and to attend to the thing at which he is looking.

As for spelling per se, the continuance of whatever teaching method is in use is all that is done. We do endeavor to decrease emphasis on extra work in this area until gross motor coordination is improved and dominance is achieved. In fact the most difficult part of this program seems to be the matter of convincing parents and teachers to wait for "hard-goods" repairs and to delay tutoring or similar remedial pressures during the growth period. In our academically oriented society, explaining that lack of ability to spell need not be cured over night — that it is not a fatal malady — is not easily accomplished.

THUS FAR, it has not been feasible for us to develop the necessary statistical data which would be acceptable in educational circles. We must, then, follow the example of the medical profession and base our indications of success on a few cases, three samples of which are summarized here.

SAMPLE CASE HISTORIES

A boy, whom we will call Bob, was referred to us as having both reading and spelling problems which had not yielded to standard remedial procedures. He was a ten-year-old Caucasian of middle-class family, the middle child in a sibship of three, the other two of whom were girls. Bob's gross motor coordination was poor, he lacked proficiency in athletics, and his conversation was often incoherent. He was right-eyed, right-eared, and right-footed, but left-handed. After three months on this program (during this period all other remedial work was discontinued at our request), he decided to learn to use his right hand, accomplished the change easily, and became sufficiently adept at baseball to join a Little League team. Within the next three months, his reading and spelling grades improved, going from a D to a B average. Better organization in his thinking was evidenced by improved coherence in communication. At this point, his mother decided that he did not need further help, and withdrew him from the program.

David was fifteen and of similar socio-economic background. School evaluations indicated that he was a potential honor student but inability to spell either on tests or when doing independent written work precluded his taking advantage of the Honors Program in his school. He was left-handed, left-footed, but right-eyed. His program included creeping and training for eye dominance with the use of a stereo-reader. He stayed with the program faithfully for about three months with an increase in both reading and spelling proficiency. At that time, he gave indications of having achieved left-eyedness. Being a very normal adolescent, he then decided he'd "had enough" and he refused to do any more work in spite of being told that he had not gone far enough for progress to be lasting. In two months he had regressed and was again failing in all written work. He then returned to his creeping and stereo-reading and worked at it faithfully for six months. At that time, he had achieved sound left-eye dominance, was able to turn in readable written work, and had been placed in the Honors Program. He is now a senior in high school and has achieved not only academic honors but standing as a top athlete as well.

Perhaps the most outstanding example is a little girl we will call Dana. Dana was not referred to us as having any kind of problem. She was the older sister of another child with whom we were working. She was a bright and musically talented eleven-year-old. Her B average at school was achieved by what her father felt to be "too much hard work" on her part. Closer evaluation revealed that she was right-handed, left-eared, and lacking in eye dominance. She was placed on the full program, from patterning through to dominance training, including the elimination of all music listening. After six months of this work, Dana had achieved right-sided dominance and she returned to her music more skillful than before her "vacation." Her A average at school was attained easily enough to allow her spare time for her music and also for the ballet ·lessons she was able to add to her schedule.

To the scientifically oriented, the only conclusion that can be drawn from the three sample cases presented here is that this program was successful in these three instances, though other factors such as motivation and extra attention were not ruled out. There are similar cases in our files; unfortunately their number is not yet sufficient to warrant statistical analysis. Until such analysis is made, we conclude: "It works so why not use it?"

REFERENCES

Delacato, Carl H. *Neurological Organization and Reading.* Springfield, Ill.: Charles C. Thomas, 1966.

Fay, Temple. "The Use of Pathological and Unlocking Reflexes in the Rehabilitation of Spastics," *American Journal of Physical Medicine,* 194 (1954), 499.

Lilly, Ellwood C., and Sarah A. "Developmental Training for the Cerebral Palsied," *Cerebral Palsy Review,* XXVI (1965), 7–8.

Spelling Problems: Diagnosis and Remediation

Shirley H. Linn

HAVE YOU suspected that poor spelling grades of some children were not so much due to laziness or poor study habits as to learning disorders?[1] You may be particularly suspicious if the youngster does not respond to extra help given by parents, teachers, or tutors. Once suspected, what can you do until the psychologist comes? Suspicion of learning disorders is not enough. Pending the psychologist's evaluation you may find it fruitful to conduct a study for clues to prove or disprove your hypothesis. These clues may be based on observation of the child as he studies, as well as consideration of the work done in his lessons. This could be considered a preliminary assessment of abilities, the findings of which can serve as a screening device for weakness in developmental areas.

Preliminary assessment of problems in spelling may be made by careful scrutiny of the child's spelling lessons and his work habits. The manner in which errors are made and the way in

which he works may reveal whether he is careless, has not studied, or if he has earnestly tried to learn to spell but was unable to achieve his goal. Of course, not one, but many observations should be made prior to developing an opinion that learning disorders exist.

Skills Necessary for Spelling.

To consider spelling as an area in which clues to learning disorders may be found, we must first look at the skills which a child must possess in order to succeed in spelling. First of all, the child must be able to reproduce in the proper order, the letters used in the word. However, the process is much more complex than this.

In order to reproduce the order in which the letters are used to make a word, a child must know the names of the letters, the sounds the letters represent, and exceptions to rules for sounds. He needs the ability to recall these symbols quickly, accurately, and to produce them on paper correctly. If he cannot do the above, what kinds of errors does he make? Does he learn any part of the word, to the exclusion of other parts? That is, he may know the first letter of every word, but it is the only part of the word he can re-

---

[1] Learning disorders, for the purpose of this paper, may be described as a developmental lag in one or more areas necessary for learning to take place in the traditional school subjects.

call correctly. Can he fuse the sound parts of words together into whole words? Does he reverse letters in sound parts? Can he remember what you have written on the board a few minutes after it is erased? Does he learn words when he hears the letter sequence rather than when he sees it? Does he appear to block out or not "hear" sounds? Can he write the correct symbol for single sounds when they are dictated to him orally? Can he identify sounds?

Diagnosis.

Errors in the above areas are clues to learning disorders. They may suggest immature or inadequate development in visual or auditory perception or association, encoding or decoding. A preliminary survey of the child's work habits may reveal indications of learning disorders, but further verification should be sought in the form of standardized tests. Developmental areas may be evaluated by such diagnostic tools as the *Frostig Developmental Test of Visual Perception,* the *Illinois Test of Psycholinguistic Abilities,* the *Wepman Test of Auditory Discrimination,* and the *Purdue Perceptual Motor Survey.*

Remediation.

Remediation depends on the disorders which are found. All too frequently, remediation techniques assume readiness of the youngster to respond. However, the child may not be developmentally ready for the level of remediation given. For example, he is not ready for phonics until he has learned to discriminate differences in sounds and to associate sounds with their symbols. He cannot accurately write letters in the proper sequence if he is still confused by left and right. Therefore, it has been found that, prior to academic achievement, children need basic motor skills and some degree of visual and auditory readiness. Both gross-motor

activities and visual-perceptual activities provide many aspects of this readiness. Especially helpful are programs by Marianne Frostig and David Horne[2] and Newell C. Kephart[3] Both of these programs contribute background information and activities to help children develop skills in these areas. Activities in these programs utilize oral directions given by the instructor, through reception of the directions auditorily, interpretation, and carrying out the instructions by motor action. When language responses are included as part of the program in action songs or similar activities, several important developmental areas may be trained at one time. Most young or mentally retarded children need more specific emphasis on language development. A new program, *The Peabody Language Development Kit* provides a well-rounded program for development of language skills.[4]

Once the child is able to achieve in the above areas, some of his difficulties in spelling should have become less severe. He should be ready for more specific training in basic spelling skills through a specialized approach. Information from the diagnostic tests should reveal strengths and weaknesses in his development. This should provide clues to the most appropriate channels to use for remediation.

It is less frustrating to use strong channels to develop weaker ones, even in spelling. For example, the child with strong visual development but weak auditory development will probably learn to spell with greater ease by

---

[2] *The Frostig Program for the Development of Visual Perception* (Chicago, Ill.: Follett, 1964).

[3] *The Slow Learner in the Classroom* (Columbus, Ohio: Charles E. Merrill, 1960).

[4] Circle Pines, Minn.: American Guidance Service, 1966.

looking or using the visual approach to learn the correct order of letters. Once he feels secure using the look-and-spell methods, sounds may be repeated orally as his eyes focus on each letter. In this way, not only is the auditory channel being used, but it is being developed in a manner that is not threatening to the youngster.

The needs of each child differ, and it is largely up to the ingenuity of the teacher to develop the appropriate approaches which will enable the child to learn. From your study of the children in your class, you may learn many things which will enrich your teaching program.

REFERENCES

Flowers, Richard M., Helen F. Gofman, and Lucie I. Lawson (eds.). *Reading Disorders.* Philadelphia, Penn.: F. A. Davis Co., 1964.

Frostig, Marianne, Welty Lefever, and John R. B. Whittlesey. *Marianne Frostig Developmental Test of Visual Perception.* Palo Alto, Calif.: Consulting Psychologists Press, 1964.

Roach, Eugene B., and Newell C. Kephart. *The Purdue Perceptual-Motor Survey.* Columbus, Ohio: Charles E. Merrill Books, 1966.

Wepman, J. *Auditory Discrimination Test.* Chicago, Ill.: Language Research Associates, 1958.

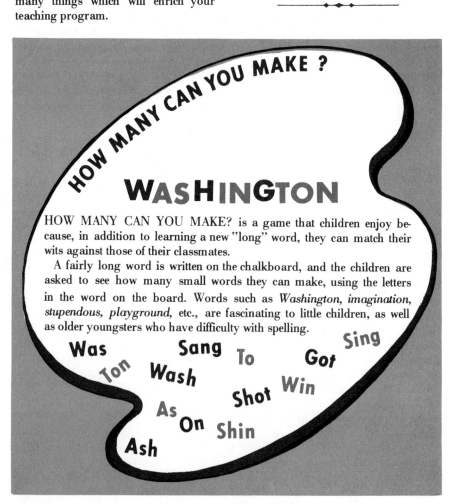

HOW MANY CAN YOU MAKE ?

WASHINGTON

HOW MANY CAN YOU MAKE? is a game that children enjoy because, in addition to learning a new "long" word, they can match their wits against those of their classmates.

A fairly long word is written on the chalkboard, and the children are asked to see how many small words they can make, using the letters in the word on the board. Words such as *Washington, imagination, stupendous, playground,* etc., are fascinating to little children, as well as older youngsters who have difficulty with spelling.

Was   Sang   To   Got   Sing
Ton   Wash   Shot   Win
As   On   Shin
Ash

Associative Memory Aids for Spelling

Ronald J. McEwan

———◆———

T HE TEACHER of spelling must be fully aware of the need to utilize as many modal input systems as possible in order to assure adequate learning by all members of a class. Too often, it seems, primary emphasis is placed upon the visual component of learning, with the resulting failure of several students. The classic approach of Fernald is, perhaps, the best single example of an integrated multisensorial approach. [1] However, except with a highly structured program and a carefully controlled population, the Fernald approach does not lend itself easily to classroom use.

At the junior and senior high school levels, most students would object to any approach to spelling which might bring direct attention to themselves as they worked out their learning problems. When attempting to teach students to use new techniques, it must be kept in mind that while it is desirable to have students utilize as many modalities as possible, the introduction of techniques which attract attention should be carefully considered.

It is with these thoughts in mind that I present the following techniques,

which I have found highly successful with many students. These learning aids are not in any way designed to take the place of traditional spelling instruction, but rather may be used as a means of organizing practice, of reinforcement, and of developing a conscious awareness of the word being learned.

A TECHNIQUE which might be called the "body movement approach" equates one body movement with each letter. For example, the word *opportunity* might be broken down in the following way:

O — Snap the fingers.
PP — Hold up the index finger and thumb.
O — Snap fingers again.
R — Rub the nose.
T — Touch the thumb to the middle finger, making a *t*.
U — Wrinkle the nose.
N — Purse the lips.
IT — Point the finger and say "it."
Y — Open the hand in an "I don't know" gesture.

Although the foregoing may seem involved and time consuming, it actually takes only two minutes or so to learn a series of gestures of one's own creation. These actions could, with some

[1] Grace M. Fernald, *Remedial Techniques in Basic School Subjects* (New York: McGraw-Hill, 1943).

slight variations, be used in a classroom without detection by other students. When studying at home, a student might move from point to point within a room or he might perform a variety of steps and actions while orally spelling a word. It is not necessary for the student to repeat these actions at school as he will probably remember his body movement and associate one letter with each movement.

Another device which is especially suitable for classroom use is to use a geometric figure or drawing. After choosing a figure and establishing a starting point, the letters of a word are placed in order at different outstanding points on the figure. Again using the word *opportunity* as an example, the pattern might be as follows:

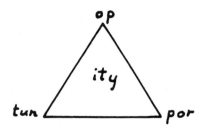

Although this aid is easy to use, it has a disadvantage in that the student must rely to a large extent upon visual memory and thus he may be easily confused.

Sometimes, while studying words, easily remembered relationships leap to mind. These associations often involve well-known aids such as recognizing little words contained within big words, relationships between parts of a large word (meaningful, perhaps, only to oneself), funny sentences which seem to make up a word, etc. Such associative devices are valuable aids and should be consciously developed, as they form the basis for word-analysis skills.

EACH of these approaches to learning spelling should be taught individually. Although it may appear, superficially, that "tricks" rather than academic skills are being taught, on closer examination it becomes apparent that these techniques are simply ways to help the student to note the sequences of letters and syllables and retain them for future use.

Teachers must be conscious of the fact that it is necessary to teach students *how* to learn. It must be remembered that some students can spell a word orally, perhaps, and yet he may be unable to recognize that word in print and be unable to write it correctly. It is therefore the teacher's job to present techniques to such students that will help them transfer each spelling word into a commodity which can be used in all ways. The associative devices described above may be helpful in achieving that end.

Improving the Language-Arts Skills of Teenage Disabled Readers

Phyllis W. Dole

READING is but one segment of the group of interrelated skills called "Language Arts." Speaking, listening, reading, spelling, and writing are all part of the communication package required in school learning and very rarely do they function totally independently of one another.

Teenage students in a remedial program not only lack reading ability, loathe writing tasks, spell atrociously, scribble illegibly, and reluctantly participate in oral communication, but, in addition, they are severely blocked because of a sense of futility and deflated self-image. In all their years in school, they have learned one thing—they are failures. Without the hope of success in school work they cloak themselves in a shroud of apathy and protect themselves from further failure experiences by refusing to participate.

These teenage students have a paucity of expressive language skills. Along with their limited ability to communicate orally, they have restricted writing skills. These are the students who in their regular classes never get anything down on paper. They receive "D" and "F" grades in social studies, science, history, and government because they do not produce written reports, daily written assignments, outside reading assignments, class reports, and other activities requiring language-arts skills. Unless such students have special help, they will drop out of school and join the ranks of untrained, illiterate youths, ill-equipped to hold a job or fulfill their own human desires.

For such severely disabled readers of junior- and senior-high-school age, the teaching of reading, writing, and spelling through the "language arts approach"—that is, learning to read the written text of their own taped utterances—has been successful at the Learning Center. Working on the principle that what you think you can say, and what you say can be represented in writing, and what is written can be read, the students have come to understand relationships of the printed word and the language it represents.

The first effort of the Learning Center program is to strengthen the students' self-image through a pattern of small successes in all learning situations. Rehabilitation begins through the skills the students already have. The students' own verbal language is used for instruction.

Reading the written text of their own spoken utterances is a stepping stone for students to make generalizations which may apply to reading the writing which represents the language of others. Though the grapheme-phoneme correspondence of English orthography is somewhat irregular, it is regular enough that the learner, from reading his own spoken material, can learn many of the discriminative functions of letters and combinations of letters to the sounds they represent.

The procedure of these lessons is as follows: Every day each student records on the tape recorder individually and privately. If the student has comments which he wishes to state about himself or his experiences, he may dictate such comments. If, however, a student is so fearful that he says he doesn't have anything to say, then he is given a picture to describe a story situation. The material is typed daily and the following day each student has his story in print. This story he reads aloud to his teacher. Difficult words are analyzed by phonetic analysis, syllabication, context cues, and other word-analysis skills.

The material the student dictates is faithfully recorded in print as he created it. Slang, idiom, personal dialect, and sentence structure are kept intact. The "personal language reading" approach is in reverse order to remedial teaching techniques frequently used in corrective reading programs. All too frequently students with reading disabilities are believed to need drill on phonics, word families, and all other word-analysis skills. These "reading tools" are taught from material of little appeal to teenagers. One of the most common complaints that teachers have when working with severely retarded teenage readers, is that there is no material interesting enough at a low achievement level for poor readers to read.

There is no problem of subject material or interest when students read their own material. The disabled reader will learn to read and spell "Honda," "girl-friend," "accelerator," "armed services," "police record," "bugs me," "split," before he reads some of our standard English, but the basic concepts can be taught from his own language patterns.

THE NEXT STEP the students take after taping their ideas for several weeks is to write their ideas. During the independent writing period they get assistance with difficult spelling words from the teacher. If the student needs a word, this is written for him on a 2"x6" slip of paper with a black grease pencil. Before the student uses the word in his writing, he traces it several times with his finger and practices writing it from memory. When he is able to write it correctly, he includes it in his written material. A dictionary file box is provided for each student. The words he has requested and studied are placed alphabetically in his dictionary word box.

At the time the student is writing independently, he is only assisted in the words he requests. When his written material is typed for him, misspellings of functional words are corrected and noted. These and the requested spelling words become his personal spelling study list.

The student's personal spelling list is continually being reorganized. As he masters words, they are deleted from the study list and new ones are added from his written material. Words are reviewed in a three-day sequence. The teacher, aide, or other students give him the trial tests. When a student can write the study words correctly for three days, the words are considered mastered. Periodically, about every six weeks, the total accumulated personal spelling list is reviewed.

The student's written material is typed as it was when he formally dictated it. This he reads the following day. At the time of rereading his material, the student and teacher discuss the ideas. Informally the student is helped to increase his skill in communication by responding to such questions as, "Can you say that another way?" "Can you add anything more about that?" "What other words can you think of that mean the same thing?"

This language-arts approach is an attempt to present a total communication package in the learning experience. The students' oral expressive language, written language, spelling power, and reading ability are extended simultaneously. The interrelatedness of speaking, reading, writing, and spelling is reinforced rather than separated into different learning tasks. For example, spelling power is enhanced by the study of word patterns and phonics during reading and, conversely, reading skills, particularly word-analysis skills, are developed by the discrimination of word parts during spelling practice.

The creative writing period and spelling practice is only part of the students' remedial program. A careful diagnosis is made of each student's reading skills, spelling power, and language development at the time he is admitted to the clinic. An individual prescriptive program is planned for a sequential development of language-arts skills. Programmed reading materials, study-skills lessons, word-analysis-skills exercises, reading in trade books for fluency and pleasure, extemporaneous speaking, expository writing, and other activities are also provided.

Using the student's own language for reading, writing, and spelling instruction does promise success. For these discouraged pupils, the first step to becoming a student is the realization that they can succeed.

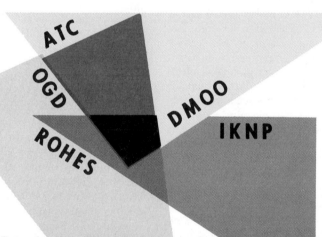

JUMBLE-O is played by jumbling the letters of words which you feel the children can spell with reasonable ease. For example, *cat* could be presented as *tca*. Write the jumbled words on the chalkboard, and say to the children, "Number one is *cat*." Thirty seconds are then allowed for the children to put the letters in the right order before proceeding to the next word, and so on.

A variation of this activity is to include an extra letter in the jumbled word, telling the children that this has been done. For example, *cat* might be jumbled as *tacy*. Be careful, however, about introducing this level of complexity before the youngsters are ready for it. It can sometimes be used as a special challenge for those children who want to try.

Two Approaches to Spelling Problems: Self-Discovery and Phonics

Jack Wahl

A Self-Discovery Approach to Spelling.

TO PRESUME that all the mistakes a child makes are related to his problem denies him the right just to be wrong. The child who cannot get his world organized from left to right is still a student, and students make mistakes. Much more than the normal student, the student who is confused as to directionality needs to know that a lack of knowledge has produced an error and not a confusion of the order of letters.

When a child misspells a word, one way to help him become aware of what he is doing wrong is to pronounce the word as he has written it. Point out the applicable phonetic rules and ask him to try again. Do not tell him how it is wrong or give him any clues except a correct pronunciation of what he has written. If the student is working on a polysyllabic word, accent the syllable that makes the most sense for the word he wants to spell. If the student is trying to spell *complete* and spells it as *c-o-m-p-e-l-e-t,* to pronounce the *o* as a short *o* instead of a schwa is only going to make it more difficult for him. The idea is to make it as easy as possible for the student to find his own mistakes by having him be-

come aware of the results of what he did as opposed to what he intended to do.

This technique is a self-discovery method, but the self-discovery is very controlled. To help the student, the word he has misspelled must be reasonably phonetic and the person doing the pronouncing must pronounce the word as closely as he can to the way the student would pronounce it.

Students seem to learn faster when the second attempt at spelling a word is placed in a column directly under the first, and the third (if there is a third) under the second, etc. Each spelling should then be pronounced as often as the student requests. Often a student will go back over three or four attempts and recognize a progression either towards the word he is trying to spell or away from it. He will then use this knowledge to arrive at a correct spelling.

IN A ONE-TO-ONE situation (one therapist to one student), with high-school students and with young adults, I have found it helpful to write the word on the chalkboard as the student dictates it, and then pronounce it as he has dictated it. Having someone else do the writing helps the student look at the word more objectively and often he makes the proper changes before I have had a chance to pronounce the original spelling.

This same process works when a student mispronounces a word while trying to read. I go to the board and write what he has said and have him compare what I have written with the word he is trying to pronounce. This turns a reading lesson into a spelling lesson, in a way, but it presents information to the student in a manner that has meaning for him. Most students quickly learn to look for sounds that are out of place, to check the number of syllables they have pronounced, to recognize reversals, etc.

The student must be made aware, from an objective point of view, of what he has done. As much time as necessary should be spent to convince the student that the important thing is the message he is trying to communicate; that what he means has no value until he has communicated it to someone else; that words that are jumbled are read by others as I (the teacher) have pronounced them, and that when they are seen that way they do not make sense – and sense is what communication is all about.

The necessity of selecting reasonably phonetic words to be used with this technique cannot be overemphasized.

Phonics for Spelling.

A TY SEVVUN per sent uv all sil-lubbuls in our langwij ar purely funnetick . . . " This statement is from *Teachers' Manual for Reading with Phonics.*[1] The complete sentence is,

"Eighty-seven percent of all English syllables in our language are purely phonetic and the words in which unphonetic syllables occur are in part phonetic."

To the child who has not yet developed sufficient visual recall to see words "in the mind's eye," more words appear to be nonphonetic than are phonetic.

I analyzed the Thorndike and Lorge "List of the Five Hundred Words Occurring Most Frequently," and made the following breakdown.[2] Seventy percent of the list is made up of one-syllable words (*a, line, your,* etc.). Fifty-one percent of these words are spelled as they sound (*rest, drop, line*). Of the words with more than one syllable, sixteen percent can be spelled the way they sound (*after, over, whether*). Only forty percent of the total list of five hundred words can be spelled as they sound.

One problem is that the sound does not always have the same graphic form. For example, in one-syllable words, the *e* sound is spelled, with almost equal frequency, *ea (eat, hear, sea)* and *ee (need, green, see)*. This is also true in multiple-syllable words where the *e* sound occurs in positions other than at the end. At the end of multiple-syllable words, we use the *y (lady, happy)*. There is, therefore, no rule for a child to follow in order to be sure of spelling the word correctly. At the ends of words, *o* sounds are made by an *o (no)* or an *ow (know),* again leaving the phonetic speller without a way of determining the correct spelling.

Some students are able to read but are unable to spell. They seem to have sufficient visual memory to recognize

[1] Julie Hay and Charles E. Wingo, *Teachers' Manual for Reading with Phonics* (New York: J. B. Lippincott, 1954).

[2] Edward Thorndike and Irving Lorge, *The Teacher's Word Book of 30,000 Words,* (New York: Teacher's College; Columbia University Press, 1944).

words, but not enough to recall the letters that make up the word. Spelling rules should be rules that apply to spelling only, not to reading – even though the two skills are related. The changes in pronunciation that have occurred since the spelling of our language was stabilized follow a pattern of their own. The conversion of sounds into symbols now follows different rules than it once did, but there is still more logic to spelling than is apparent when we look only at the phonetic rules for reading.

Rules for reading largely ignore the position of the sound in the word. It seems that the position of the sound in a word helps predict the symbol that should be used to spell it. The *j* sound at the end of a word is a good example. There are reading rules which say the letter *g* may represent the *j* sound if it is followed by an *e, i,* or *y.* The *j* sound at the end of a word is always represented by *ge (age).* This is an example of phonics for spelling.

Further investigation might lead to other predictable phonics-for-spelling rules which are not necessarily related to reading, but which meet the criteria in which the student is most interested: the production of correctly spelled words.

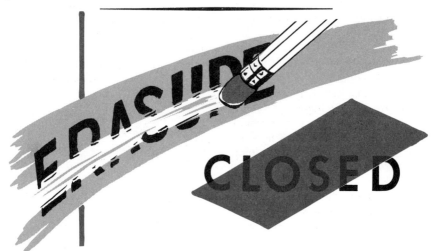

INVISIBLE WORDS is an exercise that helps youngsters to build visual memory. Write a word on the chalkboard, tell the children to look at it, then have them all close their eyes for five seconds. Have them look at the word again for another five seconds, then erase it from the chalkboard and have the children write the word.

This works well with large or small groups, can be used with "already studied" words, or words that are new to the students.

The children enjoy the variation of having the teacher write the word on the board, cover it, then asking someone to spell it orally. The word is then uncovered so that the students can see if the word was spelled correctly or not. If it was not, the process is repeated until someone succeeds in spelling the word as it is written on the board.

Accent on Spelling

Blake K. Browne

SPELLING is a skill which is based on many subskill abilities. One of the sub-areas, unfortunately often ignored, is that of rhythm. The rhythmic oral-aural language of the child is translated into graphic form as he makes the transition to higher, more complex forms of communication. This developmental transition carries with it a rhythmic basis, subtle as it may be, to adults who function comfortably with language.

We see disturbances in rhythm in children who are hypokinetic or hyperkinetic. Their gross or restricted movements strongly suggest disturbances in the basic rhythmic integration of the motor, perceptual, and cognitive areas.

In poor spellers, we notice so often that oral language is uneven, accents misplaced, and phrasing weak. When these youngsters are asked to repeat a word presented orally, they quite often have difficulty, reversing and omitting syllables. In a similar manner we observe that handwriting tends to be disorganized, the sequencing skill is weak and spotty, and the total language function seems to be out of balance.

FOLLOWING is a technique which I have found useful as a preliminary step in a total spelling program.

First, I gather the youngsters into a group seated around me. Some-times we sit on the floor, sometimes in chairs. I clap a simple pattern and encourage the children to join in with me. Sometimes it is a slow pattern, sometimes fast. Sometimes we use only our feet, sometimes our hands, and sometimes both. Sometimes we stand and let the top half of our bodies hang down and rhythmically move from the waist. Sometimes our eyes are open, sometimes they are closed. We attempt to involve the whole body.

When I see that the children are ready, we play a game in which I clap a rhythmic pattern and challenge the children as to who can repeat it exactly. With younger children this works well with rhythm instruments. Older youngsters may want to tap the rhythm out with a pencil on a hard surface.

The child who correctly repeats my pattern has his turn in creating a new pattern for someone else to repeat correctly. When a child is having difficulty, and when conditions are right, I tap a rhythm on a child's back and see if he can then clap the rhythm.

The next step in this sequence is to introduce the concept of one beat that is louder than the others. For example, instead of: *clap ... clap ... clap,* it would be: *clap ... CLAP ... clap.* Again, ample practice at this stage is necessary. This is the point at which many youngsters suddenly find themselves having difficulty. Retaining the sequence *and* retaining the point of emphasis may simply be too much to handle. If this is the case, let the children vocalize the beat by saying, "Clap ... CLAP ... clap," so that a different kind of motoric awareness is experienced.

ABOUT this time, I introduce a visual element. On the chalkboard I draw several patterns, beginning with the following:

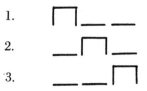

1.
2.
3.

These drawings would illustrate the following:
1. *CLAP ... clap ... clap.*
2. *clap ... CLAP ... clap.*
3. *clap ... clap ... CLAP.*

I then beat out a rhythmic pattern, asking, "Which picture goes with the pattern I clapped? Who knows?"

The transition involved in this step is obvious. We are integrating a visual stimulus with the auditory-motor pattern.

As the children become competent at this exercise, we add more visual designs to a chart which we now begin to use. We add to the complexity involved in making the correct choice of the visual pattern corresponding to the rhythmic beat.

The final step in this procedure is for the teacher to say words—slowly so that syllables are stressed. The teacher may try two possible introductions. She may start by "clapping" the name of the children, giving the primary accent to the correct syllable. For example: *BILL-y, SU-san, An-DRE-a,* and so on, clapping louder on the accented syllables as they are pronounced.

Another method is for the teacher to raise her hand on the accented syllable. For example, she would make a movement of her hand corresponding with the line as follows:

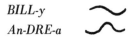

BILL-y
An-DRE-a

The teacher may also make the same kind of line on the child's back, moving her hand from left to right as she pronounces the word.

FOR OLDER CHILDREN, a technique which is enjoyable is to give them short sentences and let them see what pattern would be correct when the accent *within the sentence* is changed. For example. "WHERE are you going?" or "Where ARE you going?" or "Where are YOU going?" or "Where are you GOING?"

Because the entire body is involved and because left-to-right sequence is integrated, the children appear to respond to language patterning in spelling, as well as in reading, writing, and speaking. As with all techniques, this one is best utilized over a period of time and in conjunction with other on-going approaches designed to build competency in effective communication.

Individual Letter Reversal Reduction

Jeffrey L. Hicks

THE PRIMARY consideration of this article is the reduction of those violations of directional constancy which result in individual letter reversals within the context of whole words; for example, reading *bady* for *baby* or *dab* for *bad*. [1]

My premise is that inconsistencies in spelling can be corrected through a direct attack on reading accuracy. This article will not focus on inversions, such as reading *pad* as *bad*. That problem should be discussed in another article.

It has been my experience that specific etiological information about the student's problem is seldom available, involves more speculation than fact, and is of little direct value in planning a program for I.L.R.R. Therefore, with amelioration of the student's difficulty, I prefer to speak in terms of "symptom reduction" as opposed to claiming modifications in the causal framework of the disorder.

Where to Begin.

LET US suppose that when a particular student reads orally, he reads *b* for *d* and *p* for *q*. How should

one approach such a problem? I propose that the remedial instructor graph the incidence of such reversals in terms of number of reversals: number of reversible stimuli over X amount of time. One may thus obtain a percentage-of-error score. This percentage-of-error score may serve as a quantitative index which will change throughout the remedial program.[2] No corrective measures should be employed during this phase of the program.

The Remedial Program.

THERE ARE a number of general guidelines that should be kept in mind when designing and implementing a program for I.L.R.R.:

• Work with one letter confusion at a time. For example, if the student reverses *b* and *d* as well as reversing *p* and *q*, the remedial teacher should not attempt to correct both difficulties at the same time. Rather, one of the confusions should be dealt with at a time. This means that should the confusion between *b* and *d* be chosen as the initial focus of remediation, errors involving a confusion between *p* and

---

[1] In this paper, "individual letter reversal" will be denoted as "I.L.R." and "I.L.R.R." shall denote "individual letter reversal reduction."

[2] An analysis of errors may provide a qualitative measure of change during remedial treatment. In other words, an indication of whether of not any one specific letter confusion, i.e., *b* and *d*, occurs more often than any other.

85

q would not be brought to the attention of the student. I have found that better results can be obtained if the student has less upon which to concentrate. A program for the reduction in rate of other letter-reversal confusions should be begun only when the initial confusion has been either greatly reduced or entirely eliminated.

The teacher may feel that he is doing an injustice to the child by ignoring other types of errors. I am convinced, however, that the above approach will result in both a more immediate and lasting reduction in errors than an attempt to deal with all letter-reversal confusions at once.

• Work with one letter at a time. For example, if a reversal confusion between *b* and *d* is chosen as the initial focus of remediation, the teacher should not introduce both letters and attempt to explain the difference. Instead, one letter should be selected and a program of remediation should be designed to help the student correctly identify this letter in the context of the printed word.

• The chosen letter should be introduced through as many sensory channels as possible, i.e., visual, auditory, kinesthetic, and tactile, with an emphasis upon the student's strongest sensory modality.[3]

• Reading material should be as uniform in type of print as possible.

S ELDOM, if ever, does one find I.L.R. as an isolated problem in an otherwise adequate reader. Most often it may be viewed as one of a cluster of symptoms constituting a severe language disability. If such reversals are symptomatic of a severe language disability, it is not uncommon to find an extensive history of academic failure. Continuous academic failure often results in a lowering of the student's overall stress tolerance. For this reason, among others, I have chosen a program of remediation derived from an operant model. There are several aspects of the operant model that I find desirable for treating students who exhibit an I.L.R. difficulty:

• A minimum of instructor verbalization is necessary.

• With both correct and incorrect responses, the student receives immediate knowledge of results.

• The student can be informed of errors briefly and nonverbally, thus eliminating the emotional charge of a verbal, and often prolonged, explanation of the mistake.

Let us suppose, as previously mentioned, a particular student reverses *b* and *d* as well as *p* and *q*. If a qualitative analysis of errors indicates that one specific reversal, for example *b* and *d*, occurs more often than any other reversal in the student's oral reading, and a further analysis indicates that *b* is read as *d* more often than the reverse, the letter *b* is the logical place to begin remediation.

Having selected a specific letter, the instructor should help the student find some "associative stimulus" to aid him in distinguishing that letter from other letters differing only in directional orientation. For example, if the letter *b* were selected, the teacher might put a small spot of ink on the back of the student's right hand to remind him that the loop on lower-case manuscript *b* faces toward the spot. While reading, the student's hands should be placed on each side of the page to facilitate recognizing the proximity of the loop on *b* to the spot. It should be noted that no mention has been made to the student in regard to the spot being on the student's *right* hand. After the association be-

---

[3] I suggest administration of the *Illinois Test of Psycholinguistic Ability*, James J. McCarthy and Samuel A. Kirk (Urbana, Ill.: University of Illinois; Institute for Research on Exceptional Children, 1961).

tween the spot and the direction of the loop on *b* has been firmly established, the concept of *right* may be introduced.

AFTER the introduction of the spot on the back of the student's right hand, the student should be directed to read orally. With the occurrence of the first error involving a reversal of *b* and *d*, the instructor might tap a pencil on the top of the desk.[4] The student should then be directed to continue reading orally. With the occurrence of each subsequent reversal, the instructor should tap the pencil once. This tapping of the pencil need be only loud enough to attract the attention of the student.

In addition to this "negative reinforcement," the instructor should use "positive reinforcement" in the form of a verbal reward for each correct response of the student to either *b* or *d*. This positive reinforcement might consist of a simple "good" or "right" from the teacher.

---

[4] Other examples of nonverbal negative reinforcement are a bell or a light.

It is hypothesized that with continuous positive reinforcement (reward) in combination with negative reinforcement, the student will come to associate the tap of the pencil with an error and verbal praise with a correct response. Since the pencil tap will occur only when *b* and *d* are confused, the student will not only be informed of an error, but the correct response will also be indicated.

For a program such as the one outlined above to be successful, reinforcement must initially occur with every correct and incorrect response. Great care must also be given to the selection of the associative stimulus so that it is easily understood and remembered by the student.

This program is intended only for use in a one-to-one relationship, thus allowing the teacher to focus only on the specific student. The program, which incorporates many of the principles of operant conditioning, offers an approach to individual letter reversal remediation through which spelling may be significantly improved.

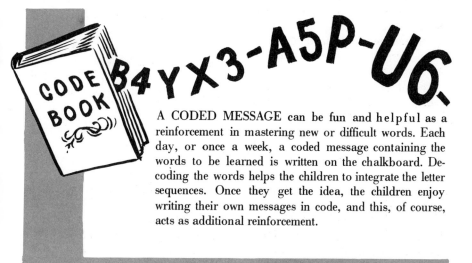

A CODED MESSAGE can be fun and helpful as a reinforcement in mastering new or difficult words. Each day, or once a week, a coded message containing the words to be learned is written on the chalkboard. Decoding the words helps the children to integrate the letter sequences. Once they get the idea, the children enjoy writing their own messages in code, and this, of course, acts as additional reinforcement.

Learning Through Three-Dimensional Texture

Eula Farnham

TEACHING the neurologically handicapped child presents a severe dilemma. Whereas repetition is vital to thoroughly imbed learning principles, the short attention span that goes with learning disability often works against this repetition. Too often not more than five or ten minutes can be devoted to a necessary basic.

I have therefore reached the conclusion already reached by others in this field — that variety is not only the spice of teaching; variety is the salt of teaching neurologically handicapped children. I find that I am usually successful with a student in direct proportion to the variety of methods I can employ to present learning opportunities. This type of teaching is the most demanding of the many approaches, and is certainly the most creative.

Techniques that help children in reading also help them with spelling, and vice versa. For example, in spelling and reading, children confuse letter forms. The technique to be described has been found helpful.

For the younger children who are just beginning therapy and for the older students with ingrained habits, I put, in the early hours of therapy, a strong emphasis on form of letters. Yet, during these same early hours, the attention span is the shortest of all.

I have used beaded letters, sandpaper letters, wooden letters, and cardboard letters — as well as letters in relief constructed of many materials. However, I wanted something different. During a dishwashing session a kitchen sponge provided the answer.

I purchased a package of kitchen sponges in a plastic bag. The sponges were of four different colors and two different sizes. The larger ones were approximately 3" by 6" and the smaller ones were 3" by 4½"; all were three-fourths inch thick. I first drew the letters of the alphabet on paper, then cut them out of the sponges. (I used ordinary large scissors to cut the sponges and found them easy to cut as long as they were still moist from the plastic bag preservative.)

The larger sponges, cut in half, gave me the small letters: *a, c, e, i, o, n, r, s, u, v, x,* and *z.* The smaller sponges provided the descenders and ascenders: *b, d, f, g, h, j, k, l, p, q, t,* and *y.* I cut *m* and *w* from the smaller sponges held lengthwise.

I MADE only the lower-case letters and used the basic forms of the manuscript printing used in the first two grades of school.

The colors of the sponges added an interest for the children, although I made no attempt to color-cue vowels and consonants because I was interested only in the economical use of the sponge material in order to obtain as many letters as possible. Color cuing would be simple to do by purchasing sponges by color instead of selecting the mixed varieties. By using four packages of sponges, I found I had surplus material from which I could cut extra letters — those that occur most frequently in our language — so that different words could be formed.

The feel of the sponges after they have dried (and they dry rapidly, so they should be cut immediately after opening the plastic bag) is a rough texture on all surfaces. This makes tactile learning possible. Because it is three dimensional, the student can feel all around the letter. Sometimes, for example, I pass a letter to a child under the table and he must identify it by feel alone.

Rightness and leftness has to be established with many of the letters before the child can correctly identify them. The b - d - p - q flipover becomes obvious to the child and therefore he must get the letter "set" in his mind from feel alone. He then must place it on the table in the proper position to be read.

As a variation, I have the child place his hands behind him and I hand him the letter to be identified. This gives a different perspective to the form. He then brings the letter forward and must identify it visually when it is placed on the table.

WITH A CHILD who is totally unaware of the differences between the b and the d, I have him describe how he is turning the letter about under the table in relation to the center or midline of his body. In what direction does the circular portion protrude to form the b (right or left)? In what direction does the circular portion protrude to form the d (right or left)?

If the child holds the letters in his right hand, the straight portion of the b would be under his index finger and the other fingers would be encircling the rounded part. For the d, the circular part would be under the curled thumb and first two fingers and the straight portion would be under the last two fingers.

Again, using the same idea, the reverse of these positions would be true if the letter is placed in the left hand.

With the b and p reversals, the straight portion of the letter, under the right hand, either extends up so that the forefinger is straight, or it extends down toward the wrist.

These "intellectualizing" exercises are done both with the eyes open and then closed.

The t and f and the n and u lend themselves to this same kind of analysis. The rightness or leftness of each letter can be investigated if difficulties arise as to which direction a letter must be placed to be read correctly.

TO FURTHER emphasize the form and visual shape of a letter, I give the student a shallow container of poster paint and a large sheet of newsprint. By dipping the sponge in the paint and printing b all over the paper, at the same time saying the name and the phonetic sound of the letter, the child gains experience with the letter through several senses. When printing the b, the child must hold his index finger on the straight portion of the letter in order to get an even print. The other flip-forms of the letter b are tackled in the same way.

The washability of the sponges after using them with paint (and after being handled by grimy boy hands) is an aid to the teacher. The sponges must be laid out flat, after squeezing out excess water, in order that they assume the proper dry form. When dry, the sponges can be stood on edge easily if there is a bit of flat area left at the bottom of the round letters. The letters that project below the line in printing cannot be stood on edge, but this very fact impresses the child because the letters sit in relationship to a line of type.

By wetting a sponge, imprints are possible on a blackboard, especially a chalk-covered blackboard. A complete washing of the blackboard can be done after the session. (One should be sure that the blackboard is the type on which water can be used.)

By double printing the *b* on both the newsprint and blackboard, using it as a *b* and a *d,* the relationship of the two letters becomes apparent. The four flips of the *b* can be done in four different colors so that the child sees what the form can do in four different positions.

THIS TECHNIQUE has many interesting and artistic variation possibilities. For example, powdered window cleaner in paste form can be used on glass for holiday decorating. Interesting designs can be made with single letters, or a repetitious all-over pattern may prove to be surprisingly artistic. Another idea is to have the child print the letters of his name on heavy art paper. These letters can then be cut out and attached to one another by strings to form a mobile.

The possibilities of this method are endless, but the important thing is that it does provide a variation for holding the interest of children with a short attention span while helping them to learn to discriminate form of letters.

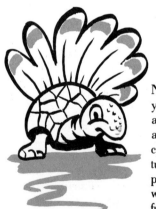

NEW ZOO is a gamelike approach to spelling which young children enjoy. The names of two familiar animals are blended to make a new word. For example, *turtle* and *turkey* could become a *turkle;* a *lion* and a *goose* could become a *gion.* The children can then draw pictures of the new "animals." The exercise offers an opportunity for the youngsters to use sounds in different ways, and the pictures that follow are often delightfully funny.

Auditory Fusion as a Spelling Technique

Lyle Putnam

A NUMBER of spelling techniques are also useful in building word-attack skills. The specific technique to be described was developed to help children improve their reading as well as their spelling abilities. It has proved beneficial to many children with language deficits, particularly when there is a wide gap between reading/spelling age and chronological age. The ability to blend or fuse sounds is a basic one. It leads to fluent, sequential language; but training is a gradual process and cannot be hurried.

To assist children with fusing word elements, I have them play a number of oral word games. At first, I introduce listening games for auditory sequencing when there are three or four minutes before a recess, or as a "quieting-down" time following a particularly active lunch period. I have found these games useful, for some children, as an auditory reinforcement for left-to-right sequence of letters within a word.

On the chalkboard I draw three broad lines as follows:

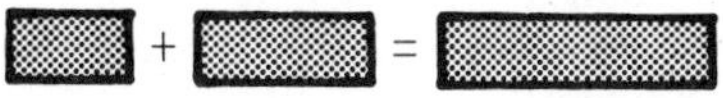

I say, "I'm thinking of a flower – a *r-r-r-r* . . . *ose*." As I pronounce the *r* sound (not the letter name), I point to the first short line on the left-hand side. As I say *ose*, I point to the second line. I then point to the line on the right-hand side. "Now, who can give me this – the name all put together?"

While this exercise may sound and look easy, it is surprising the number of children who have difficulty with it. To help such youngsters, I sometimes begin with names of children in the class. For example: "I am thinking of the name of a boy in our room. *B-B-B-B-B* . . . *ill.* Of whom am I thinking ?"

When this technique is being introduced, it is important that the teacher point to the lines (illustration above) in sequence (from left to right) as the sounds are being given. For some children, the visual association is not readily apparent; then suddenly they realize that the large line on the right side is the combination of the two sounds.

For younger children, or even some older youngsters, it is sometimes helpful to illustrate the concept of fusing by locking two pieces of a puzzle together, or by having two jars of colored liquid and pouring them together to get a third color.

The best results are achieved when reinforcement is given with words in the speaking and listening vocabularies of the children. For word building, new words may be introduced as the children become more facile in handling the technique.

After a period of time, as the children become quite skillful, I have them move their hands across the surface of their desks to get the feel of the movement from left to right as the word is being fused.

IF THERE continues to be a need for integrating the ability to fuse word elements with the visual representation of the word, I prepare a tape in which one-syllable words are pronounced as described above, that is: "*C-c-c-c . . . ome; l-l-l-l . . . ook; g-g-g-g . . . o*"; and so on. The student is given a sheet of paper with words listed as follows:

1. look   come   corn   cow
2. stay   look   by   book
3. toe   got   go   gone

As he listens to the tape, the student is instructed to circle the words he hears. At the end of the tape, the student's paper should be checked immediately. If he misses any of the words, the tape should be played again and the procedure repeated.

When this approach is first introduced, the teacher should select words to be listed on the sheet that are obviously different in appearance. For example: *look, come, done, rang.* If the child seems comfortable with initial lists of this sort, lists in which the words are more similar may be introduced. For example: *look, book, hook, nook.*

A small group of students, using earphones, can work together in practicing this method. One student may be appointed the monitor for starting, stopping, and rewinding the tape.

It should be remembered that the purpose of the technique is to build in the child an auditory anwareness of left-to-right sequence through a physical awareness. The method should be used along with other activities designed to build the child's total language efficiency.

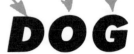

Do Only Good → DOG

FIRST LETTER ONLY is a brief mental exercise in letter discrimination which the children enjoy. From a prepared list, the teacher explains to the students: "I am going to spell a word by giving you a sentence. The mystery word is made from the first letter of each word in the sentence." The sentence given might be, for example, "Sue owns many eggs." The answer, of course, would be *some*. At first the sentence may be written on the chalkboard. Later, as the children become more familiar with the technique, the teacher may dictate it.

Make It Attractive

Sandra Winkler

————————◆————————

MUST we always have children use a black lead pencil on white, lined paper for writing and spelling? While the effect of this tradition on spelling is debatable, using color in spelling is fun, different, and motivational for children. It adds a dimension that is new and stimulating.

Either through your local school district, or from the local five-and-dime, inexpensive sets of colored pencils can be obtained, one set for each child in your class. Also available are pads or paper in different colors; or you can, instead, have the children line construction paper – enough to have a supply on hand. (This is a good activity for use of the ruler and a straightedge and for hand-eye coordination.)

You can vary the approach. One day every child might be given yellow paper for spelling and be allowed to use any pencil he or she wishes for any one word. On another day, you might allow the children to choose the color of paper they want to use, but instruct them to use only a dark pencil.

The results of these exercises in color are quite attractive and can, if the children wish, be displayed on the class bulletin board. Some children like to save them in their spelling notebooks. Occasionally, the children like to draw a design or cut scallops around the edges of the paper. (Again, a good activity for hand-eye coordination.)

A chalkboard is always fascinating to children and although they are standard equipment in most classrooms, too often the children themselves seldom have an opportunity to write on them.

I have had excellent results with poor spellers, utilizing this valuable teaching tool. A supply of good-quality colored chalk should be kept on hand. It is available in a wide variety of pastel colors from art supply houses.

Let the children go to the chalkboard and write their spelling words in any colors they wish. Rather than restricting each child to a small area, limit the number of children at the board at one time, allowing each one plenty of space. Let them write any three words they wish, three times each, and then have them return to their desks so that others may have a turn.

I have often found it helpful, when a child is studying a word which is particularly difficult for him, to have him write the word in one color and the "tricky" part in red. (Red signifies "caution.") The act of putting one pencil or piece of chalk down and picking up another at the problem point is an aid to the child's memory, as is the color emphasis in the visual representation of the completed word.

Occasionally, as additional motivation, I have the students use light green paper. When a word is learned, the child is allowed to write it on yellow paper and pin it on the class bulletin board.

INTRODUCING new and imaginative ways for children to practice difficult spelling words not only reduces the resistance to working on the problem words, but it also helps the child to retain the words through visual memory. Following are some simple techniques that seem to be effective.

For "rainbow writing," two or three different-colored crayons or colored pencils are held together with a rubber band and the child writes the word with which he is having difficulty. As a further stimulus, he might write the word several times, using different combinations of colors each time. Sheets of colored art paper may be used for additional eye appeal.

Another idea is to give each child a large, primary-sized crayon and have him, using the broad side of the crayon, "draw" the troublesome word on a large sheet of white art paper. With water colors, he then paints over the entire surface of the paper with a variety of light colors. The waxed area, where the word was drawn, resists the water colors and thus stands out from the background with a strong visual effect.

The next method is one which the children find particularly delightful. The child is given a piece of heavy tagboard and some slow-drying glue. He first writes the difficult word lightly in pencil on the tagboard. The next step is to have him squeeze a line of glue over the penciled lines. He then sprinkles glitter over the entire sheet. When the glue dries, the surplus glitter is shaken off, leaving only that which has stuck to the glue. The word which has been such a source of annoyance to the youngster is suddenly before him – a sparkling work of art.

When you liven up a routine spelling class with color, you may be surprised that your youngsters have suddenly found that spelling is something to which they look forward.

SDRAWKCAB BACKWARDS

EMAC GAME

BACKWARDS is a good game for developing visualization ability along with basic spelling skill. Select a word which you believe all of the children should know and spell it backwards. For example, you might spell *to* as *o-t*. The children are then asked to spell the word as it should be.

Initially, it may be necessary to allow the children to use pencil and paper, but the goal is to have them learn to manipulate the symbols mentally. From simple, two-letter words, gradually progress to longer words of four or five letters.

Using Word Forms for Spelling Competency

Bernard Bailey

A TECHNIQUE that is especially helpful with other than young children, although it has been used successfully with them also, is one which involves building of spelling efficiency through a recognition of form. This method seems to have a particularly successful impact with youngsters in the twelve- to fifteen-year-old range.

I introduce the approach by printing a word on the chalkboard and then, using the side of the chalk, I block the word out in very straight lines so that the word itself is almost obliterated. For example, the word *park* would become ▰▰▰.The students get the idea quickly with a few examples.

The next step is to hand out dittoed sheets with words printed on them in letters that are approximately three-fourths inch high. This encourages the children to make well defined corners around the words. I ask them to do the same as I did with the words on the chalkboard.

If the children are young, they enjoy using crayons instead of their pencils. Even some older students enjoy using colored pencils, so it is a good idea to have them available.

Continue this procedure for a period of several days. Observe the reactions of the students. Look for an awareness of shape and form. The children will begin (when they see the outlines for *like* and *tale*, for example) to comment, "Hey, these two are the same!"

When this awareness begins to emerge, the children are ready to move to a more advanced level of the method. I hand out sheets containing approximately twelve items such as the following:

1. ▰▰ park   hike   wink   look
2. ▰▰ feel   have   half   want
3. ▰▰ how   now   see   when

To begin with, the teacher can be very generous with time allowed for completion of the sheets. Later, the amount of time should be reduced. The student is requested to circle the correct word. At this stage the ability to read the word is not important. The students should, however, be able to recognize the correct word without resorting to drawing forms around each word on the line. If a youngster is unable to do this, or is slower than his classmates, he should be dropped back a step.

FOR REINFORCEMENT for slower students, I use a set of cardboard forms which I have precut. The student is then given three-by-five-inch cards with individual words printed on them. He matches the forms to the words by actually placing the form over the word. He may even trace around the form as a check for accuracy.

When I note that the students are making progress in recognizing the form which goes with a word, I again move into a highter level of visual response. I give each student a dittoed paper such as the following:

If the two are the same, leave them alone and go on to the next line. If the two are different, draw a line through them.

1. park   park
2. in the house   in the horse
3. has a car   has a jar
4. strange   strange

Exercises such as this, once again, should not emphasize the actual reading of the words or phrases. The focus is to be placed on the visual recognition of likenesses and differences.

If students are having difficulties with these exercises, reduce the level of complexity by using shorter words or even by using simple forms such as the following:

1.
2.
3.

As the children begin to develop a building-in of word forms as a retentive skill, the transition can be made away from forms into words themselves. At this stage, I still do not stress oral recognition—only visual recognition of likenesses and differences. I have done this in the following way:

Circle the two in each line that are exactly the same.

1. park   bark   hark   park
2. when   what   that   what
3. live   hive   have   have

A variation of this exercise is to ask the students to circle the two words that are different. It is a good idea to alter directions on activities such as this, particularly when you are trying to build awareness of both likeness and difference.

When the youngsters have progressed through this series, they will not necessarily have become skillful spellers, but they will have become more aware of the variation of forms and details within words by building retention. They will have become overtly conscious of differences among words. They will be more ready to actively participate in the mechanics of learning to spell comfortably and efficiently. They will have a more solid foundation.

Time Charts for Poor Spellers

Helen S. Barnette

THIS STUDY was made to find a method for helping underachievers recognize the merits of home study. The hypothesis was that such pupils could improve their spelling by studying the assigned lesson twenty (or more) minutes for five evenings before they were tested.

Selection of Pupils.

From the class rolls of all eighth-grade sections, I listed every pupil who had a report-card grade in spelling of C or below for the second six weeks of the school term. No other criterion was used in selecting the seventy-five participants whose intelligence ranged from 72 to 120 on the *Otis Test of Mental Ability.* The median I.Q. was 101. It is interesting to note that eighteen of the participating pupils had IQ's of 110 or higher and that fifteen had I.Q.'s of 90 or lower. On the spelling section of the *Stanford Achievement Test,* the median grade level for these students was 6.9 in September, and 7.9 in May.

Procedure.

Arousal of a desire for spelling improvement served as motivation for the experiment. Likening this device to a crutch, the teacher suggested that it be used only until the pupil strengthened his study habits. Instruction continued as for the other pupils and the same as during the previous grading period. Briefly, the following plan was used:

Friday

• Pupils independently overviewed the new word list to find unfamiliar words. Meanings and pronunciations were checked.

• A detailed class discussion was held of specifics as they applied to the words in the list:

1. Variant definitions.

2. Structural analysis of less familiar words: (a) Phonetic spelling as in a glossary. (b) Accent. (c) Other acceptable pronunciations and/or spellings.

3. How the spelling of roots and/or derivatives varies or is similar to the word to be learned for the week.

4. Word origins: (a) Singular and plural forms (alumnus, alumna, alumnae). (b) Characteristic endings (bureau, beau, cafe, coupe). (c) Greek or Latin stems (bi-ology, sten-o-graph-er).

• Development of techniques for remembering spelling of difficult words.

• Assignment of study helps from the text.

Following Thursday

• Pupils corrected their homework papers.

97

- Time was allowed for questions.
- The teacher dictated words; the pupils wrote them.

- Accuracy was checked. The pupils sometimes checked their own work, sometimes the teacher checked the papers, and at times the pupils exchanged papers.

- A summary was made of perfect scores, common errors, etc. This was done at the beginning of the period on Friday when the teacher checked the papers.

In addition to learning to spell the words, all pupils who were habitually misspelling twenty percent (or more) of their weekly assignment were asked to note the study time spent each evening. Three different formats for the study chart were tried during the experiment. Figure 1 shows the most successful one.

FIGURE 1

To the Parent or Guardian of _____

Because we know that certain activities contribute to the learning process in spelling, we make homework assignments with this in mind. To help improve his spelling, we suggest that the pupil pay attention to the items listed. He should record his study time each evening after he has learned 4 or 5 words, have it verified by a signature on Wednesday, and bring this sheet to class with the homework every Thursday.

Items needing *special attention* are indicated by a check mark.

1. Spend a minimum of 20 minutes each evening studying the assignment.
2. Distribute study periods over several evenings instead of spending an hour or more at one sitting.
3. Use study method demonstrated in the front of the text.
4. Learn the pronunciation and meanings of every word he learns to spell.
5. Complete homework assignments accurately.

NUMBER OF MINUTES SPENT STUDYING SPELLING

UNIT ____   T ____ F ____ Week-end _____   M ___ T ___ W ___ Total _____
Parent's Signature _____   Score ____

UNIT ____   T ____ F ____ Week-end _____   M ___ T ___ W ___ Total _____
Parent's Signature _____   Score ____

UNIT ____   T ____ F ____ Week-end _____   M ___ T ___ W ___ Total _____
Parent's Signature _____   Score ____

UNIT ____   T ____ F ____ Week-end _____   M ___ T ___ W ___ Total _____
Parent's Signature _____   Score ____

On Wednesday evening one of the parents was requested to sign the time chart. On Thursday the pupils turned in the chart with their homework. When someone forgot his chart or brought it unsigned, his test score remained uncredited until he brought the chart signed as requested.

At the end of five units of words, a review test of thirty-five items was given. Twenty-five of the test words were taken from the current five units, while ten of the words were review from units studied earlier in the year.

Interpretation of Results.

• All except two of the seventy-five pupils who participated in this study showed some improvement over their spelling record for the preceding six weeks.

• The greatest improvement was made by a boy (I.Q. 90) who correctly spelled fifty-three more words during the study. He showed an average improvement of 6.4 words per week, plus an improvement of fifteen words on the twenty-five-word six-weeks review, plus an improvement of six words on the ten-word review of the semester's work.

• One boy who spelled ten less words correctly during the study had flu and was absent from school for eight days. He also had a job after school.

• A scatter graph of the increase in the number of words spelled correctly showed the following during the six-week experiment:

Median improvement of 10 words out of 100 assigned to average groups for weekly tests 10%

Median improvement of 10 words out of assigned to superior groups for weekly tests 8%

Median improvement on six-weeks test of 35 words was 6 words . . . . . . 17% (This would indicate that retention was definitely strengthened.)

Median improvement on total words spelled 14

• The average overall improvement was 14.35 words during the six-weeks period, or 12+%.

• Pupils using the charts reported a median average of fifty-eight minutes per week spent in studying spelling.

• Applying the rank-order method to study the variance between gain in words spelled correctly and number of minutes used for study, I found a correlation coefficient of .05, which is of negligible significance.

During the following six-week period no charts were required by the teacher. Several pupils asked about charts and it was suggested that they keep their own. No one did. Scores dropped noticeably.

Time charts were again distributed by the teacher and used by the pupils for the next grading period. Again the scores rose.

Several parents commented favorably on the use of the charts. The boy who showed the most improvement remarked, "The time chart doesn't teach me to spell, but it reminds me to learn my words.

Borderline spellers seemed to exert additional effort so that they wouldn't need to use this crutch.